S0-ARN-542

energy ecstasy
and your seven vital chakras

by bernard gunther

chakra paintings by
philip kirkland

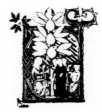

The Guild of Tutors Press

1019 Gayley Avenue   Los Angeles, California 90024

copyright ©1978
by bernard gunther
all rights reserved including
the right of reproduction
in whole or in part in any
form, published by
the guild of tutors press/ic books
1019 gayley avenue
los angeles,
california, 90024

ISBN–O-89615-OOO-3
library of congress
catalog card number
77-87416
manufactured in
the united states
of america

contents

to
the ultimate
supreme
infinite
love
bliss
peace
that is
bhagwan
shree
rajneesh

acknowledgement

heart
full
felt
feeling
thanks

for the inspiration of
Bhagwan Rajneesh

for the dedication of
Jack Schwartz*
Philip Kirkland
Phyllis Lathers
Barbara Nash
and Dede Smith

*i wish to extend
special credit
and appreciation
to my friend
and colleague
Jack Schwartz
for teaching me
some of the theory
and exercises
found in this book

a book about
human energy,
the energy body
and 7 energy centers.

it explains the way
these centers affect
the balance harmony
of the endocrine glands,
the autonomic nervous
system and the
whole psycho/physical/
spiritual organism.

the practical aspects
of the book consist of
various forms of light,
color, sound, meditation,
mantras, joyous songs
and chants.
it includes breathing,
cleansing, awareness,
visualizations and
subtle touch methods
for inner/outer integration.
the techniques act as a
bridge between the
right/left hemispheres,
the conscious and
the unconscious, to
provide a method for
self-diagnosis, self-
regulation and healing.
these pleasurable exercises
will increase energy,
creativity, relaxation,
health and well being
leading to the cultivation
and continuous renewal
of a state of stable,
flowing unity with one's
self, the world,
and others.

the game we play
is let's pretend
and pretend
we're not pretending

we choose to forget
who we are
and then forget
that we've forgotten

who are we
really

the center
that watches
and runs the show
that can choose
which way
it will go

the I AM
consciousness
that powerful
loving perfect
reflection
of the cosmos

but in our attempt
to cope with
early situations
we chose or were
hypnotized into
a passive position

to avoid punishment
or the loss of love
we choose to deny
our response/ability
pretending that
things just happened
or that we were
being controlled
taken over

we put ourselves
down
and have become
used to this
masochistic posture
this weakness
this unsureness
this indecisiveness

but we are
in reality
free
a center
of cosmic
energy

your will
is your power

don't pretend
you don't have it

or you won't

stop playing
poor me

either you will
or you won't

be willing
to express
your will power
in a skillful
loving manner

remember
by saying
to your SELF
I will
not be
swallowed up by
undesirable thoughts
feelings
or circumstances

I refuse
to identify with them
I AM
not these thoughts
feelings or circumstances
I will not let them
dominate me

I AM
now always
in each situation
as fully free
as I allow myself
to be

you are the sun
not the moon
nor the clouds

no matter what
the weather
you are always
shining

the new age
is now

it's about time
bliss
timelessness

balance
energy

infinite consciousness

moving through
to a deeper source

leaving our
preoccupation
with the past
our fear
of the future
our overstressing
the rational mind
superficial sex
excessive competition
consuming material
power games
our bitching
and negativity

to realize

who we are
and what it is
we want

the quest

the question
the questionnaire

who are you

a body

a mind

a role

a goal

you are
consciousness

a loving powerful
eternal soul

with the quality
of an observer
who has
thoughts
emotions
sensations

you have
a physical body
but you are not
that everchanging
form

you have
feelings and
emotions
but you are not
these
fluctuating patterns

you have
a mind
but you are not
this panorama
of ideas
pictures and thoughts

the body
feelings and thoughts
are all impermanent
changing instruments
of experience
perception
action and reaction

you are
an always
constant center
of pure radiant
energy consciousness

I AM
SATORI

all else
is trans/satori

for
all you are
you see

is energy

different degrees
of speed
density
intensity

chains of linking
atoms in space
patterns
in the delight dance
of everchanging matter

go look
somewhere else
for subject matter
for what does
the subject matter
for all matter
is subject to
other matter

and it

really

doesn't

matter

or it
only matters
for a while

for energy
is the sun
earth air sea
you me

chemistry
electricity
your body
breathing
circulation
sensation
impulses
thoughts
words
images
sounds
colors

this paper
book
chair
floor
to ceiling

unlimited life

consciousness

vibrating
everywhere

in various
states
solid
liquid
gas jewels
invisible molecules
finding their
temporary place
in endless
space

you are
a series
of energy fields
in a field of energy
the eternal play
of the gross subtle
shadow light
night and day

exchanging
interchanging
rearranging
itself
in the evolution
dream called
life

formless free
the cosmic energy
delightfully
created form
and will continue
to reform
in subtler
and subtler form
until it
again returns
to its former
formless form

the following
ancient/modern
energy system
to be presented
in this book
is a model
a guide map
that can assist you
to enhance

your awareness

being

creative
spirit

mind
body
dance

sit down,
close your eyes
and imagine
a white light sun
6 inches
above the
top of your head.
see the bottom
of the sun open
pouring white
light energy
down toward
the top of your head.

open your head
and let this
soothing light come
slowly into
and through
every space,
muscle, nerve,
bone, organ, cell,
atom and molecule
of your head.
now, let this
warm nourishing energy
flow through
every inch of you;
into your neck, shoulders,
down your arms
and out your hands.
let it pour down into
your torso: chest,
stomach and back;
through your hips,
lower legs, feet
and out your toes.

let the energy move throug
every inch of you.
then , close
your fingers and toes
and let your body being
be filled to overflowing
with this soft,
bright, soothing light.
let it completely saturate
the inside and cover
the outside of you.
take your time,
as much as you need.
then, let the image
of the light fade;
experience how you feel
and open your eyes.

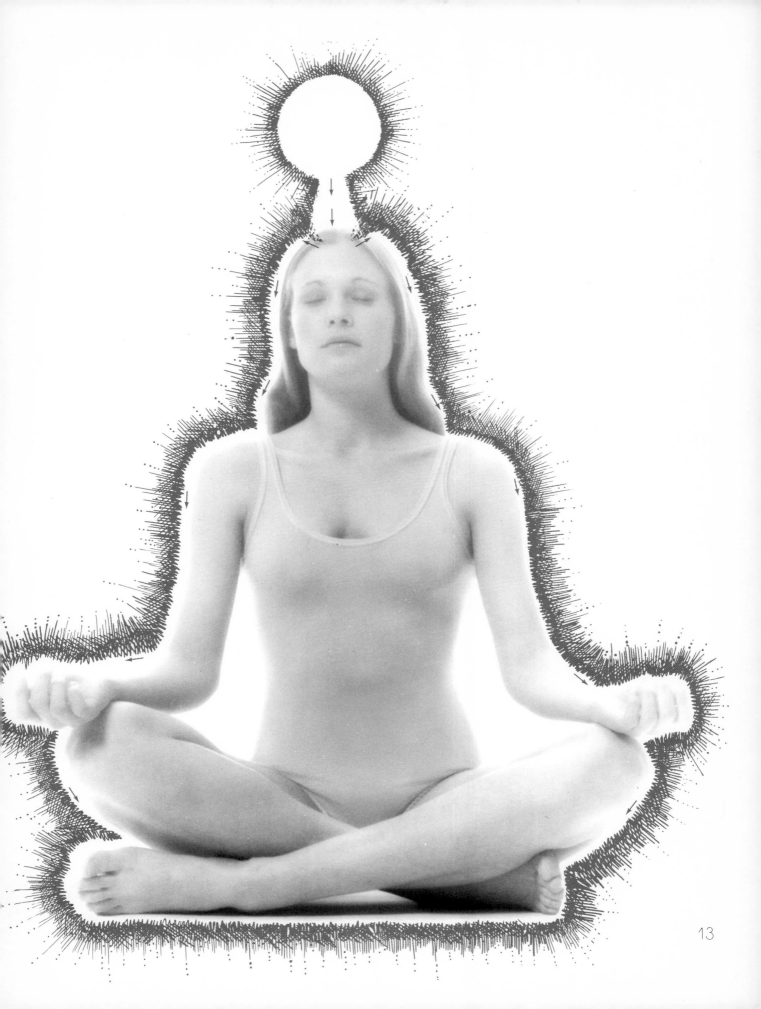

there is
a series
of fine,
subtle
energy bodies
within,
permeating
and emanating
outside of
the dense
observable
physical body.

according to psychics
with extrasensory perception,
the physical,
emotional,
mental organism
gets most of its
primary energy
from invisible rays
which come down
into the organism
through minute openings
in the top
of the head.

these rays
entering the head
may be single colored
or dual in nature.

each color,
its quantity
and positon,
whether it forms
the inside
or outside
of the ray,
will affect
the unique talent,
vitality,
disposition, personality
character,
and behavior pattern
of the individual.

as this energy
comes into the head,
it is filtered
and reflected
downward
through seven etheric
energy centers
called chakras.
these energy wheels,
or lotuses,
are located
just in front
of the spinal column
at the following locations:

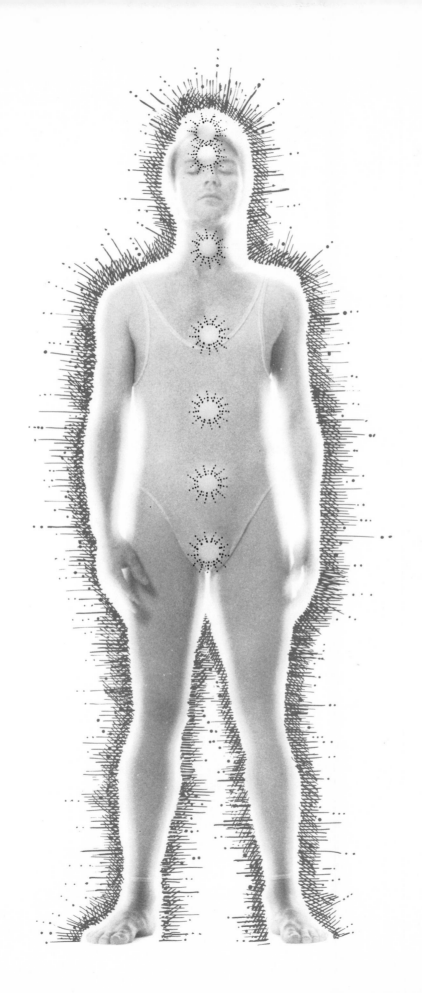

the crown center
at the top
of the head
is to be found
at an intersection
created by two lines,
one coming down the head
through the fontanel
at the upper back
of the head,
the other
through the middle
of the forehead.

the brow center
is found
at the first
cervical vertebra.

the throat center is
at the third cervical,
and the heart center
at the first thoracic.

the solar plexus is
at the eighth thoracic,
the spleen center
at the first lumbar,
and the sacrum
just above the coccyx.

as this suble energy
comes into the head,
it moves down
an extremely fine
invisible stem
located in the center
of the spinal cord.

as it filters down
through each center,
it becomes more
and more dense
so that when it
reaches the chakra
at the base of the spine.
it is relatively heavy,
very low,
slow frequency.

here it mixes with
a dense, dormant
earth energy
known in yoga as
kundalini (serpent power).

according to many different
eastern and western,
ancient and modern
ways of liberation,
it is the task
of the individual consciousne
to mix, raise,
balance, and refine
this energy force
and direct it upward.

as this ascent occurs,
the various energies
are blended and transmuted
creating a variety
of experiences
and profound changes
in awareness.

the ultimate goal
is not only
to raise this
vertical energy,
but to appropriately open
and balance
each of these
horizontal centers fully
in a flowing harmony
up, down, in, throughout
the whole
total mind/body/soul
our system.

these seven centers
are related to
and have a significant
effect on
the endocrine glands.

and these
ductless glands
ultimately affect
the whole organism.

if the flow
through these
energy wheels
is excessive,
blocked,
or disrupted
by inadequate
or undue activity,
the corresponding
endocrine
will be affected.

these glands
of internal secretion
along with
the nervous system
are the master
internal
controlling,
balancing,
and self-regulating
system
of the unified
mind/body.

the slightest imbalance
in these areas
can cause fluctuations
in minute
but extremely

powerful hormone secretions
that enter directly
into the blood stream
creating subtle
instantaneous changes
in mood,
appearance,
relaxation, respiration,
digestion,
initiative, and intelligence.

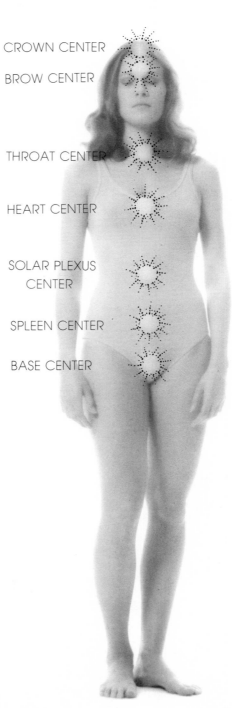

CROWN CENTER

BROW CENTER

THROAT CENTER

HEART CENTER

SOLAR PLEXUS
CENTER

SPLEEN CENTER

BASE CENTER

the power of this
internal energy system
can be related
to the chi energy
in t'ai chi
and the ki force
in akido and karate
as well as to
the basic principles
of acupuncture.

the acupuncture points
and their meridians
can be thought of
as the tributaries
flowing from
these seven rivers
of light.
if these centers
become blocked
or disharmonized,
these subtle estuaries
become unbalanced
causing symptoms
and malfunctions
in weak
or symbolic areas
within the organism.

according to chinese
and occult medicine,
all physical, emotional,
and psychological illness
is the result of
an improper balance
or an interruption
of this vital energy flow.
if this delicate
natural balance is restored,
the person once again
becomes a unified center
of well-being
bliss, health, harmony,
wholeness.

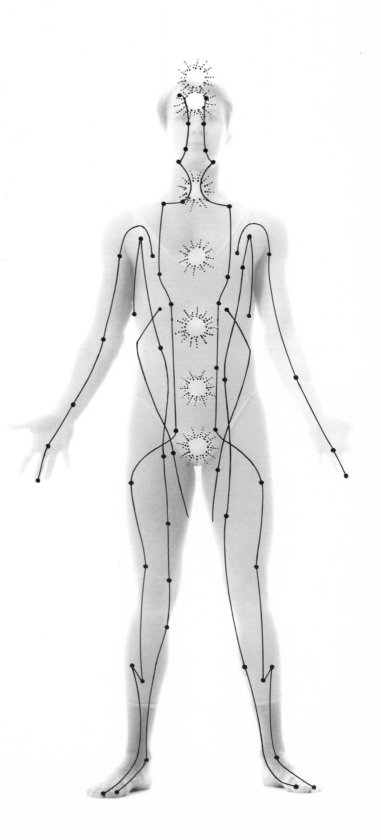

each of these centers
has its own
function, color, sound,
and symbolic form.
by understanding
these forms
of condensed energy,
each of these wheels
can be
appropriately
cleansed, opened,
and balanced.

basic exercises
for this purpose
will be found
throughout this book.

various systems differ
in the number,
location, function,
symbol, sound,
and color
of the centers.

the method
used in this book
is based less on tradition
and more on actual
visual, experimental,
and experiential evidence.

the first center,
the root chakra
located at
the base of the spine,
is the seat
of the physical life force,
kundalini.
classically
the function
of this center
is said to be
concerned with
basic existence
and survival.

for us, the function
of the base center
is to influence
sexual activity,
regeneration, and creativity.
this chakra
affects the sex glands,
ovaries and testes.
It is responsible for
the sex drive,
reproduction, and the
secondary sex characteristics.

the transmutation
of this procreative energy
can be used
to enhance all forms
of creative activity,
personal growth,
health, healing,
intuition,
and intelligence.

influenced by
the planet saturn,
earth is the element
of the first lotus,
the square
its symbolic form,
and lead its metal.

smell is the dominant
sense of the base chakra,
its color is red-orange,
and the sound vibration
of the root center is
LA.

the second center
or spleen chakra,
located halfway between
the pubis and the navel,
is usually considered
the center of
sexual activity.

in our system
it is the center
for cleansing,
purification,
and health.
its endocrine function
is connected with
the liver, pancreas,
and spleen,
glands that influence
metabolism,
digestion,
the detoxifications
of poisons,
immunity to disease,
and the balance
of blood sugar.

influenced by the
planet jupiter,
water is the element
of the second center,
tin its metal,
and taste
its dominant sense.

the symbolic form
of the spleen chakra
is a pyramid
with the capstone removed;
its color is pink,
and the sound
of the second lotus is
BA.

the third center,
the solar plexus,
located just
above the navel,
is the center of
emotion and power.
this third chakra
influences the adrenal glands
which profoundly affect
the sympathetic nervous system,
muscular energy,
heartbeat,
digestion,
circulation, and mood.

excessive use
and overabuse
of adrenalin
due to constant stress
produces various physical
and psychological symptoms
including ulcers,
nervous disorders,
and chronic fatigue.

influenced by
the planet mars,
fire is the element
of the power chakra,
iron its metal,
and sight
its dominant sense.

the symbolic form
of the third center
is a circle,
its color is kelly green,
and the sound
of this lotus
is like the emotional cheer
at a football game,
RA.

the heart chakra
is the center center,
the source of boundless
love and compassion,
rather than
one dimensional
sexual or
sentimental romantic passion.

located in the center
of the chest,
the heart lotus
when fully opened
expresses unconditional love
for spirit,
consciousness,
and every
level manifestation
of creation.

the fourth chakra
influences the thymus gland
located in the center of the chest
just behind
the upper breast bone.
the main function
of the thymus
in adults
is the proper utilization
of the
amino-competence factor,
that aspect
of the body
which helps create
immunity to disease.

it is interesting to note
how open, loving people
are usually hearty,
and how our culture's
competitive emphasis
makes people hardhearted,
susceptible to
heart disease.

influenced by
the planet venus,
air is the element
of the love lotus,
copper its metal,
and touch
the dominant sense.

the symbolic form
of this chakra
is the equilateral cross,
its color is yellow-gold,
and the sound vibration
of the fourth chakra
is the two-syllable sound
YM (Ya-Mm).

the fifth chakra
is located
in the throat.
it is the center
for creativity
and self-expression.

the throat center
influences
the thyroid gland
which affects the balance
of the entire
nervous system,
metabolism,
muscular control,
and body heat production.

this center is called
the gateway to liberation
because it leads
beyond the physical/
emotional planes
and into the astral spaces.

influenced by
the planet mercury,
ether is its element,
and hearing,
the dominant sense
of this lotus,
with mercury as its metal.

the symbolic form
of this chakra
is a chalice
(the integrated
physical/emotional body
becomes the holy grail).

its color is sky blue,
and its sound vibration
is the joyous delight
expressed in
the act of creation
HA.

the sixth chakra,
the all seeing
third eye,
is located
just above and between
the brows,
in the center
of the forehead.

here is the source of ecstasy,
extrasensory perception,
clairvoyance, clairaudience,
heightened intuition,
and the paranormal powers.
in ancient egyptian paintings
and statues,
one sometimes sees
a pharoah or initiate
with a snake figure
coming out at this point
in the forehead.
this is symbolic
of that person having raised
the latent serpent energy
to this level
which is also known as
christ consciousness.

classically,
the sixth center
is said to influence
the pineal gland,
but in our system,
it relates to the pituitary
which in sequential order
is located below the pineal.

the pituitary gland
is the master control center
of the mind/body
affecting to some degree
all of the other endocrines.

beyond the senses
and the five elements,
the sixth center
is influenced by
the sun and the moon;
its metals are gold
and silver,
and its symbolic form
is a six-pointed star.

indigo, a pure midnight blue,
is the color
of the brow center,
while the sound vibration
of the third eye
is related to the utterance
one makes when finally
reaching a deep insight
or experiencing the solution
to a baffling problem;
that sound is
AH.

the crown chakra,
or thousand-petaled lotus,
is located in and around
the upper skull.

in mystic lore,
when the lower energies
are balanced,
refined, and raised
to this region
known as cosmic consciousness,
unconditional enlightenment
beyond name,
form,
thought,
or rational experience
takes place.
it is this
highest frequency
that is the source
of the halo
that surrounds the head
of spiritually evolved beings.

the seventh center
influences the pineal gland
which medically
seems to have no function,
though the ancients
thought it was
the seat of the soul.

beyond the five elements,
mind, senses, and form,
the inexplicable state

realized at this center
is unmitigated
bliss/rapture.

total unity
with the source,
the mystical,
transcendental,
timeless,
changeless
experience of I AM,
pure being,
without subject or object
(i and my father are one).

the color
of the crown chakra
is purple,
and its symbolic form
is a lotus flower
(with its roots in the mud,
the dense energies
of the base center,
its stem in the water,
the emotional energies
of the torso,
but its blossom,
untouched by the water,
fully open
to the energy
of the sun).

the sound vibration
of this center
is the total amalgamation
of all sounds,
OM.

the human aura

is the energy field
that surrounds the
material body.
it is the sum total
of the energy given off
by the centers;
it is the glow
of part of the aura
that is pictured in
kirlian photography.

the aura has been mapped
into seven bands
or layers by observers
and is distinguished
as follows:

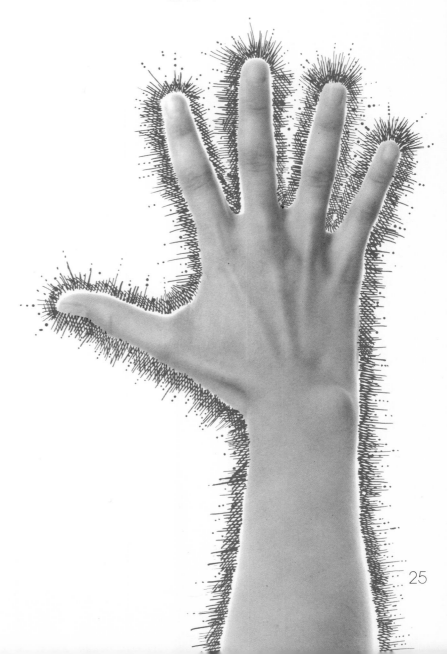

the ovum is
a one-eighth inch
blank space
between the physical body
and the first color emanation.

the first layer,
the health band,
radiates bluish white
under most normal conditions.
if a person
has a health problem,
there will be localized dark spots
related to
the origin of the problem
or there may be
a color change
in the whole aura.

the next space is
the emotional band
which reflects
the feeling level
of that person's experience.

next we find
the mental band
that deals with
the individual's
thought patterns.

the fourth
or para-conscious band
has to do with
intuition and
extrasensory power,
(most people are
totally unconscious
of the fact
that they have
these outer layers).

the fifth or
causal layer
corresponds to personal karma
(previous action).

the sixth layer,
or spiritual band,
is related to soul evolution.

the seventh,
or cosmic band,
connects with
universal consciousness.

each of these bands
radiates different colors
of varying intensity.
these emanations
can be seen
and read
by sensitives
who can tell
a person's personality makeup,
state of health,
emotional disposition,
mental attitudes,
abilities, and aptitudes,
as well as past problems,
difficulties,
and tendencies.

through the use
of this sensitive vision,
individuals can be advised
of future directions
and trends
in personal,
interpersonal,
and transpersonal
development.

(my own experience
is that i feel
rather than see the centers
and can,
with this ability,
tell which of the chakras
are open
and which are
partially blocked.)

by experiencing
the condition of the centers
and knowing their functions,
it is possible
to get a relatively
clear idea
of what a person
is holding back;
for example,
people with power problems
will be somewhat closed
in the solar plexus,
while a person
with congestion
in the throat center
will often not be
expressing himself
or his creativity.

the implications
of this sensitive sight
for health, creativity,
and optimal functioning,
as well as for
therapeutic diagnosis
and treatment,
are obvious.

according to practitioners,
a great many people
have this gift
and can be trained
to see and feel
in this way.

and so we move
out of the nineteenth century
piscean materialism
and into twentieth century
aquarian energy space,
entering a new age
where individual progress
is directly related
to group evolution,
a time when what has been
esoteric
will become exoteric;
the invisible
will become visible
in the age-old rediscovery
of the subtle,
indivisible truth
that radiates out
from within.

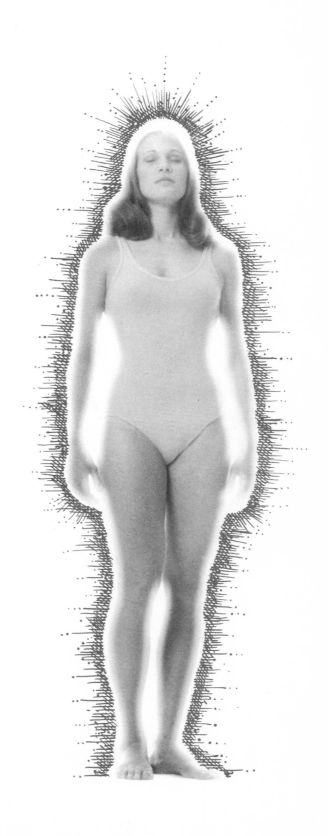

we are all
points of light
and as we link
light up
we are

turning the world
into a star.

chapter 1
ENERGY MEDITATIONS

the universe,
your existence,
is a vast whole,
a hologram.
every energy,
feeling, thought,
quality, desire,
and its opposite,
time and no time,
is there
around you.

all any being/
situation
can do
is to
touch/stimulate
that place
that is always there,
an aspect
of that
which is
all around you.

for every thing,
past, present, future,
person, possibility,
is going on,
all existing
at the same time.

your being,
moving through
every simple/
complex plane,
joy, bliss, pain,
with and against
the grain.

but our conditioned
ego identification
and our biological
social filters

organize and linearly
distort our awareness
so that we
are usually
only conscious of
one or some
aspects at a time.

the figure or figures
that are
most homeostatically
or symbolically rewarding
emerge from the
background of totality.
for example,
when you are feeling
very depressed,
low down,
discouraged,
courage exists
within you.
it is there,
but you are only
narrowly aware
so that you don't
experience it.

in this
constricted situation,
your consciousness
is largely
identified with
the negative side,
and you are not
in contact
with your being,
that deep,
centered perspective
which is beyond
any limited association
and which has
the power to
encourage you.

now drugs,
of course,
provide one way
to open more doors,
to become more open,.
to perceive more,
but you come
to depend on them,
and the price
is too often
inconsistent motivation,
concentration,
and functional preciseness.

so the direction
we are looking for
is to be more
perennially centered,
accepting and observing
who/what/where
we are at each moment,
to be
loose, natural, and easy,
more meditatively,
attentively alive.

fully aware,
totally there,
for every activity
or quiet space,
as much as possible,
in touch/harmony
with our
full perspective.

this kind of
wholesomeness
can be realized
through continuous
self remembering
and by moving
out of the hole
where the identification
perspective
is deceptively shallow,
narrow, one-sided,
and limited,
and into wider,
higher states of energy,
consciousness,
where the ability
to see/experience/feel
expands
until you are
able to fuse
with the whole.

this process
can be accelerated
through constantly
witnessing your behavior
and using
the exercises
and meditations
found in this book
to keep your
energy universe
cleansed, harmonious,
vital, and balanced.

by gradually quieting
and disidentifying
with desires,
wonderings, and distractions,
this focused force
can keep you
continuously aware,
and through the building
of this identification
with the self,
you can learn to
merge/be
compassionately

nonattached,
unified,
and disidentified.

like the open sky,
not getting carried away
by passing clouds,
thoughts, feelings,
and pictures.

but clearly
able to be,
to watch,
and enjoy your movie
without getting caught
in it
so that you can
transform,
transcend, and end
the illusory,
partial
point of view
which is the cause
of almost all
of your suffering.

first clap your hands
at various speeds
for about 30 seconds,
then put your hands
facing palms up
on your knees.
close your eyes
and experience what's happening
in your hands,
not just the slight stinging
on the surface,
but what's happening
in the center of the hands.
let that feeling
flow up your arms into your body.
let it flow
wherever it wants to go.

now open your eyes.
place your hands
in front of you,
two or three inches apart,
then very slowly
move them back and forth,
closer and farther apart.
the motion is like
playing an accordian.
don't go too close together
or too far apart.
feel what's happening.

in most cases
you will be aware
of warmth
or a feeling of
magnetic attraction
or resistance
between the hands.
you might feel any
one, two, or all three
of the above.

your body is a battery
of water cells.
your arms are the
positive and negative cables.

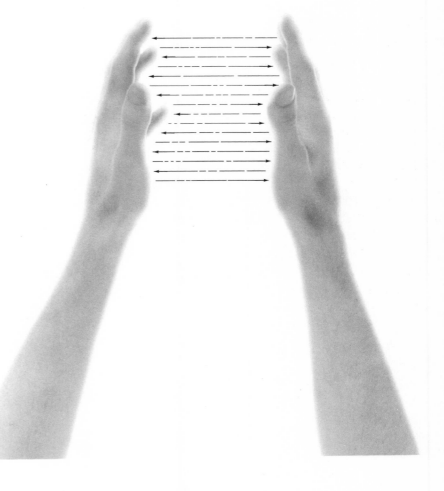

psychic energy

to increase
the energy between
your hands
use thought power.
with your hands facing
each other,
feel the energy
and then think warm.
imagine a red hot force
between your hands.
after you feel the heat,
change that force
between your hands to resistance
by imagining
a powerful current
that keeps your hands
from coming together.
then experiment:
use light or sound
between your hands,
and experience
the results.

this is a simple experiment
in mind over matter.

in tibet, initiates were taught
to use their mental concentration
to the point
where they could
sit outside naked
in the middle of winter
and melt snow.

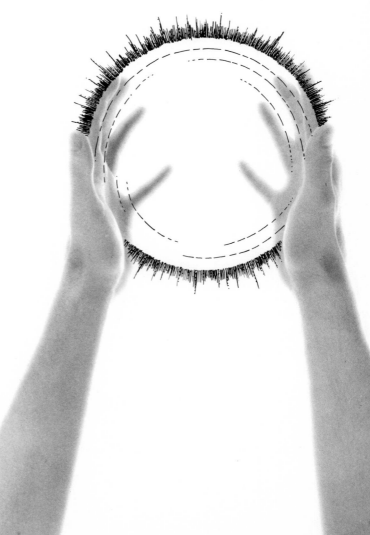

energy in/hand/sir

to balance and harmonize
the emotional energy
in the solar plexus,
place the left hand
flat on the area
just above the navel,
the right hand on top
of the left.

to balance, stimulate
and harmonize the energy
in the heart center,
place the right hand
flat over the center of the chest,
the left hand
on top of the right.

to balance and harmonize
the relationship between
the solar plexus and heart,
place the left hand
over the solar plexus,
the right hand over the heart.

to balance and enhance
the energy within the spinal cord,
sit on your left hand;
make sure the center of the hand
is under the bottom
of the spine.
the right hand
goes over the back top
of the head.
try switching hands
and experience the difference.

keep each of these positions
for 30 to 60 seconds,
or as long as desired.

these hand positions
are especially useful
when you are upset,
over-emotional, or under
excessive tension.

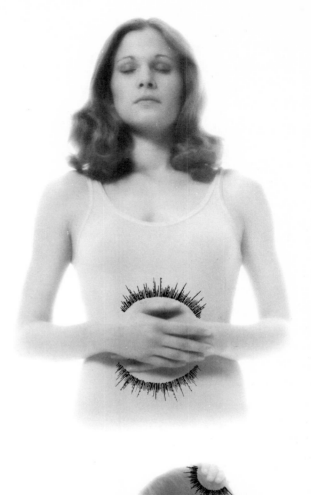

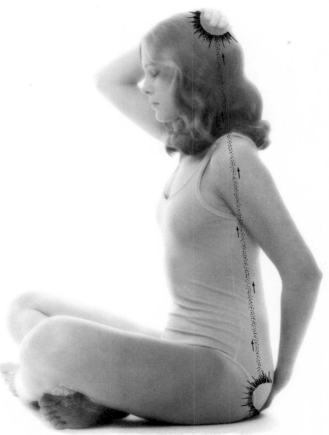

increasing energy

sit comfortably with your
back and neck straight,
eyes closed.

create a glowing pink light
at the level
of your heart center.
hold it there
for a slow count of 9.
next, see a glowing pink light
just above the top of the head.
hold it there for a
slow count of 15.
then visualize a pink light
surrounding your entire body.
you are sitting
in the middle of that light.
hold that image around you
for a slow count of 12.

then create a radiating blue light
at the level of your throat
and hold it there
for a slow count of 9.
next see a radiating blue light
just above the top of the head.
hold it there for a
slow count of 15.
then visualize a blue light
surrounding your entire body.
you are sitting
in the middle of that light.
hold the image around you
for a slow count of 12.

now create a glowing white light
at the level of your forehead
and hold it there
for a slow count of 9.
next see a glowing white light
just above the top of your head.
hold it there
for a slow count of 15.
then visualize a white light
surrounding your entire body.
you are sitting
in the middle of that light.
hold the image
of that glowing light
for a slow count of 12.

after, experience how you feel
and open your eyes.

this process can calm
as well as energize.

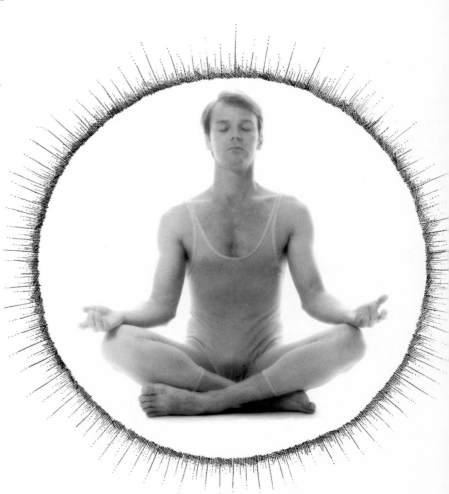

cleansing meditation

sit comfortably
with your back
and neck straight,
eyes closed.

imagine a 6-inch sun
6 inches above your head.
this sun is radiating
warm, white-light energy.
see the bottom of the sun open
pouring this purifying
white light down
to the top of your head.
now visualize at the upper head
a closed lotus flower
which slowly and fully opens
as the sun energy
pours in and downward,
saturating, purifying, balancing,
harmonizing and energizing
the crown center.
repeat this process of
slowly opening the closed flower
and allowing the light
to permeate through
the brow, throat,
heart, solar plexus, spleen
and base center.

next, connect and combine
these centers
one to the other
by seeing and feeling
a stream of light energy
flowing from one to the other;
from the base to the spleen,
spleen to solar plexus,
solar plexus to heart,
heart to throat,
throat to brow center,
brow to crown center.
then take a moment or two
to experience how you feel.

next visualize your physical body
as a closed flower.
slowly it opens fully
to the light
which pours in and downward
cleansing and balancing,
energizing and harmonizing.

next, within the open
physical form,
see a closed flower
that represents the emotional body.
feel that flower slowly opening fully
to the cleansing white light.

now see a closed flower
that represents your mental body
and experience it opening
to the purifying light.

then open the closed flower
that represents your spiritual body
and let it be saturated
by the sun light.

next blend and fuse these bodies
one to the other:
the physical to the emotional,
the emotional with the mental,
the mental with the spiritual.
take a moment to experience this.

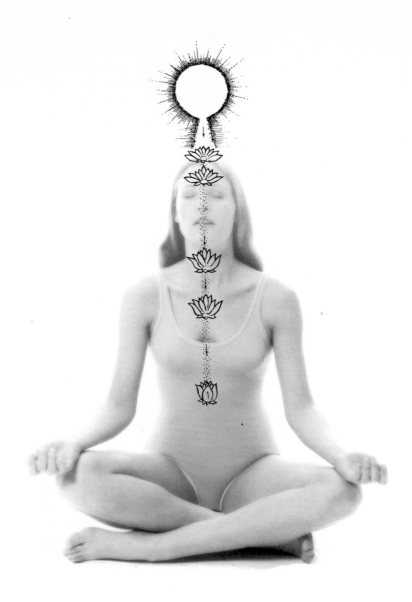

now blend these aspects
of the mind
one to the other:
the unconscious to the conscious,
the conscious
to the superconscious.

after, take a few moments
to experience the effects
and then open your eyes.

become free of the
psychophysical/emotional fatigue
toxins and debris
that accumulate
during the day.

then see in your mind's eye
a closed flower
that represents your
unconscious mind.
let the light pour in and
and downward
clearing, cleansing,
balancing and harmonizing.

next see a closed flower
that represents your
conscious mind
and allow it to open
to the incoming light.

next see a closed flower
that represents your
superconscious mind
and watch it open
to the healing light.

forehead/solar plexus/heart

sit comfortably
with your back
and neck straight,
eyes closed.

focus your consciousness
on your forehead.
keep it there
for a few moments
until you experience
that area warm and alive.
now move down
to your solar plexus
and hold
your awareness there.
next bring it up
to your heart
and spend some time there.
then move back
to your forehead,
again, back to the solar plexus,
and up to your heart;
forehead, solar plexus, heart.
repeat this cycle slowly
at least 3 times.

then, if you wish,
continue at the same speed,
increase the speed,
or reverse the order
for a period of time
until the heat/energy
is strongly felt
in these centers.

balancing and enhancing
the connection
between the mind,
love and emotions.

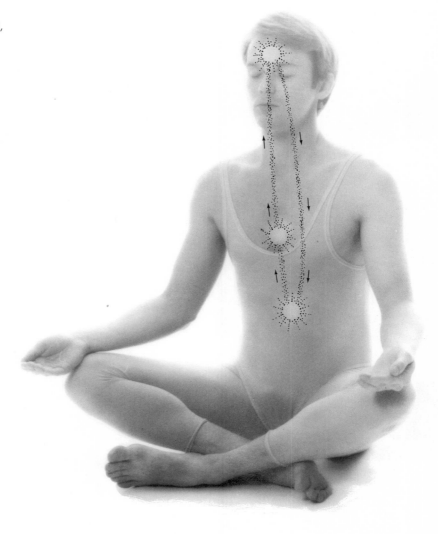

energy charge

lie on your back on the floor,
take a deep breath
and make the sound AH
as loud as possible.
continue to make the sound
as long as your breath lasts.
repeat this process
2 more times.

next undulate your belly
sucking your belly
in and out for 30 to 60 seconds,
allowing your upper body
to move as much as it can
while still lying
flat on the floor.

now, take a
deep breath
and make the sound OH.
do this over a cycle
of 3 breaths.

then do the
belly/upper body undulations
again for 30 to 60 seconds.

repeat this entire process
3 to 9 times
and experience the results.

a practical way to get
the energy moving at the
start of the day or when you
experience tension
and fatigue.

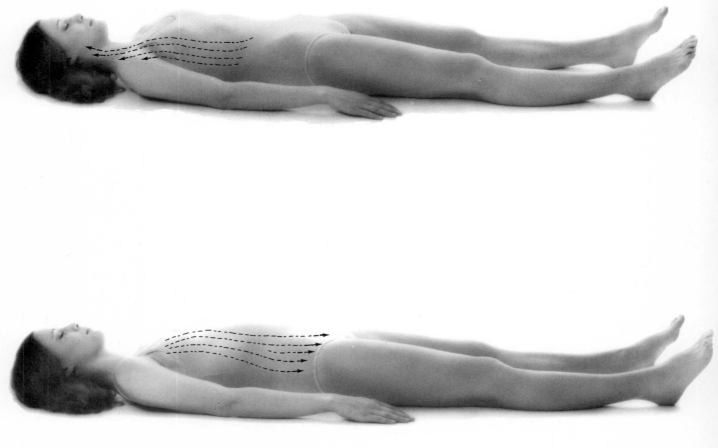

universal light

close your eyes
and create a 6-inch
white-light sun
6 inches above your head.

see the bottom
of the sun open,
pouring liquid-like
white-light energy
into you.
fill and feel
your entire body aglow
with this flowing,
soothing, bright-light energy.

now see that glow grow
so that it encompasses
the room you're sitting in.
next let that emanation
move out to include
the neighborhood around you.
then let it open up
to include the city
you're living in,
expanding even more
throughout the entire state,
opening up even wider
to include the entire country,
then the whole hemisphere,
the entire world,
the solar system,
the galaxy,
the universe.

see yourself as a dynamo
of light
in a universe of light.
as long as it feels right.

then let go,
experience how you feel,
and open your eyes.

the more you
open up to
and share the light,
the more it will
move through you.

be light
head
heart
id

chapter 2
BALANCING YOUR CENTERS

balance
is flexibility,
steadiness,
stability,
the ability
to flow
back and forth
with agility
in unlimited possibility.

without falling
too far off,
dis/ability.

for balance is
a basic key
to being
bliss/health/harmony.

the difficulty
is that
most of us
live as if balance
is jumping
from one extreme
to the other.

like riding the ends
of a teeter-totter,
we become involved
in excessive binges,
hopping
back and forth
from depression
to elation,
boredom to excitation,
love/hate/frustration,
forgetting
that real lasting balance
is within,
an alive neutral point
at the fulcrum
of your being,
and that

extreme
extremes
are extremely

painful.

the central, nervous system,
brain and spinal cord
offer us
a profound perspective.
for this self-balancing system
and can be divided
into two polar parts:
the sympathetic
and the parasympathetic.
the first of these halves
operates during emergencies,
contracting in readiness
for fight or flight,
while the latter is
related to dilation,
expansive regeneration.

at their extremes
these poles can
analogously represent
the hyperactivity
of the united states
and the inertia
to be found in india.

like india and america,
they are symbolic
of both a personal
and world-wide excess
that creates chronic
physiological/psychological/
ecological imbalance,
tension, irritation,
dissatisfaction, and disease.

these behavioral extremes
are further confused
and compounded
by the use and abuse
of language.

our verbal symbolic systems
take over and run us,
and we get lost.

instead of identifying
and cultivating
our conscious,
our being,
we become attached to
and identified with
our roles, desires,
fantasies, concepts,
and beliefs,
associating and
reacting to them
as if they were real.

like pavlov's dogs,
we salivate to a bell
even when no food
is around.

we become nervous,
tense, and angry
at imaginary dangers,
mentally creating
physical, psychological,
and eventually
depression,
fear and rejection,
the need for protection.

our minds
tyranically rule
and deceive us
to the degree
that we are unable
to tell the difference
between actual
and symbolic reality.

most of the time,
thoughts, emotions,
the past, future,
dominate our consciousness,
disrupting and dissipating
our energies
so that we miss
the unique
reality satisfaction
of simply being
with what is
now.

we seldom allow time
to stop,
to expand,
to transform,
to care for ourselves
and one another.

even sexual intimacy
has become an
ego status game,
turning a gentle
love, playful,
regenerative,
biological pleasure
into a tense,
orgasm-oriented,
goal orientation,
with all the frustrations,
malfunctions,
and seeming threats
of an actual
survival situation.

the alternative
we can choose
is to consciously be
accepting, centered
aware, natural, and easy,
compassionately
nonattached,
and totally involved
in discipline
and spontaneity.

learning to constantly
observe and experience
with sensitivity.

not going
too far off balance
so that we can regain
our own balance.

like a tightrope walker,
if we don't go
too far off
in any direction,
we won't fall down
and need
someone else
to pick us up.

using observation,
skillfull will,
focused energy,
constructive thought,
visualizations,
and chakra meditations
to continually
reestablish
and keep balance.

feeling and experiencing
the active/quiet,
passive/expressive cycles
that move
through the mind/body.

continually allowing
new ideas,
feelings,
and patterns that
let us be
appropriately
open,
clear, and easy,
in rest
and activity,
acting with the center
rather than
stereotype reacting
from the periphery,
responding totally
to the everchanging flow
to that
which actually is.

sound centering

sit comfortably with your
back and neck straight,
eyes closed.

take a deep breath
and make a low
deep OM sound.
let this vibration
encompass the entire area
from the base of the spine
to the solar plexus
including the belly.
repeat 2 more times.
experience the effects.

next make a
medium range OM sound
vibrating in the area
of the etheric heart in
the center of the chest.
repeat 2 more times.
experience the results.

then make a
loud, high-pitched OM sound
vibrating throughout the head.
repeat 2 more times.
experience how you feel.

this simple exercise
is most rewarding
when you are feeling scattered
and are willing to
take the energy/time
to return to center.

...hakra breathing

...t comfortably
...ith your back
...nd neck straight,
...yes closed.

...nhale white light energy
...hrough your mouth
...o an 8 count
...nto the base center.
...old it there
...or a count of 4.
...s you exhale
...hrough your nose
...o a count of 8,
...ee the center glow.
...old the glow
...ithout breathing
...or a count of 4.

...gain, draw white light energy
...hrough your mouth
...o a count of 8
...nto the base center.
...old it there
...or a count of 4.
...ow, as you exhale
...hrough your nose
...o an 8 count,
...end the energy
...p the spine
...o the spleen center
...nd see it glow there
...ithout breathing
...or a count of 4.

next, inhale white light energy
through your mouth
to a count of 8
into the base center.
hold it there for 4.
as you exhale
through your nose,
raise the energy
1 count
to the spleen center
and 7 counts
to the solar plexus center.
hold for 4
without breathing
and see the
solar plexus glow.

now, draw white light energy
through your mouth
to a count of 8
into the base center.
hold it there
for a count of 4.
exhale through your nose,
and raise the energy
1 count
to the spleen center,
1 count
to the solar plexus center,
1 count
to the spleen center,
and 6 counts
to the heart center.
hold for 4
and see the heart glow.

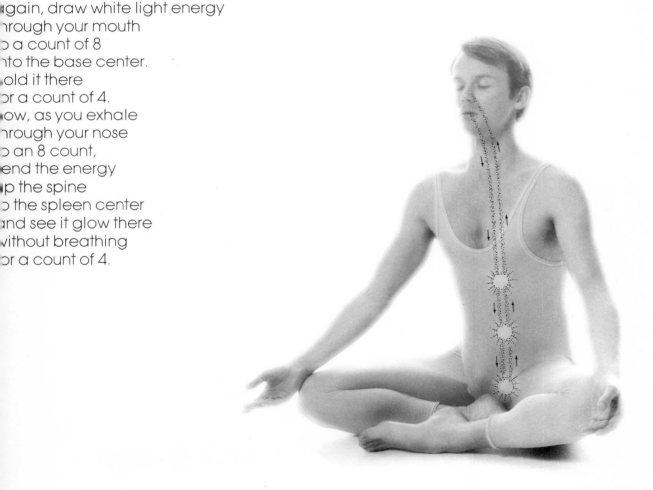

inhale white light energy
through your mouth
to an 8 count
into the base center.
hold it there for 4.
exhale through your nose
and raise the energy
1 count
to the spleen center,
1 count
to the solar plexus center,
1 count
to the heart center,
and 5 counts
to the throat center.
hold for 4
and see the throat glow.

inhale white light energy
through your mouth
to the count of 8
into the base center.
hold it there for 4.
exhale through your nose
and raise the energy
1 count
to the spleen center,
1 count
to the solar plexus center,
1 count
to the heart center,
1 count
to the throat center.
and 4 counts
to the brow.
hold for 4 without breathing
and see the brow glow.

inhale white light energy
through your mouth
to the count of 8
into the base center.
hold it there for 4.
exhale through your nose
and raise the energy
1 count
to the spleen center,
1 count
to the solar plexus center,
1 count
to the heart center,
1 count
to the throat center,
1 count
to the brow center,
and 3 counts
to the crown center.
hold for 4
without breathing
and see the crown glow.

repeat this exercise
a total of 3 times
and experience
how you feel.

this activity
raises the level and amoun
of energy in the body
as it balances the centers.

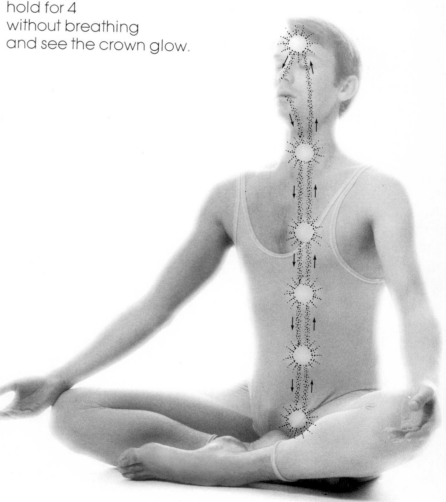

colors through centers

sit comfortably
with your back
and neck straight,
eyes closed.

visualize
the color red-orange
radiating in the
base center.
after 15 seconds,
see it as a
red-orange searchlight beam
radiating light beams
forward from the body,
radiating from the
back of the body,
radiating to the
right from the body,
radiating to the
left from the body,
radiating downward
into the floor,
radiating upward
to the sky.
see it shine
in all 6 directions
at once.
now let that
emanating light
become white,
and hold this image
for 10 to 20 seconds.

repeat this sequence
in each of the other
6 centers
using these specific
colors in each center:

spleen	pink
solar plexus	kelly green
heart	yellow-gold
throat	sky blue
brow	indigo
crown	purple

each time, after radiating
the specific color
in all 6 directions,
let that color
become white light.

sounds of centers

take a deep breath
through the mouth
and make the sound
LA
as you make this sound
let it vibrate
at the base of the spine.
on the next breath
as you make the sound
LA
see a red orange light
radiating/vibrating
at the base center.
on the third breath
make the sound
LA
and see a white light
as you vibrate the sound
in the base center.

repeat this sequence
changing the sound
color and location
that is appropriate
for each chakra:

spleen
sound BA
color pink

solar plexus
sound RA
color kelly green

heart
sound YM (Ya Mm)
color yellow-gold

throat
sound HA
color sky blue

brow
sound AH
color indigo

crown
sound OM
color purple

always end each procedure
with white light in
the chakra you are working.

this exercise is for cleansing
the lungs, expansion of
the breath, balancing
and energizing the centers.

a less complicated version
of this exercise
is just to make
the designated sound
in the individual center
3 times
without the color.

this simple form
can easily be done
while performing
an activity,
even driving a car.

draw the energy centers

meditate on each center
one by one.
try to feel, smell,
taste, experience
each in turn.
then, using colored
felt pens,
paints or crayons
draw that center.
examine the drawing
and move on
to the next center.

when you have drawn
all 7 of your centers
place them on the floor,
in order,
one above the other.
then meditate on the whole
experience the energy
you feel from them.

periodically
repeat this exercise
to make contact
with growth changes.

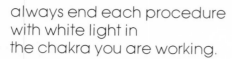

all of these
chakra exercises
can have
a powerful effect
on you.
be aware
of your reactions
and do not
overdo.

the following
symbolic chakra exercises
are some of the
most powerful
this writer has
ever experienced.
they involve the integrated
use of color, breathing
and symbols
to cleanse and rebalance
all of the centers.

as you do the process
the colors and feelings
you have
are an indication
of the state
your centers are in
at that specific time.
black or dark browns
are usually indicative
of blockage and disharmony,
while bright colors
suggest some congestion
and lack of balance.
soft, whitish colors,
(bluish-white, greenish-white,)
mean clearing and flow
while gray, white or opaque
are signals that
the center is clear.

the idea of these exercises
is not to make
the lighter or whiter
colors appear,
but to accept what emerges,
and then, if necessary,
work with the center
until that clarity
appears on its own.

how you feel
after each sequence
is as important
as the color you get.

in fact,
in the final analysis
when trying to diagnose
whether a center
is clear,
let your feelings
take precedence
over the color.

if a center does not clear
after doing the exercise
3 times,
repeat the sequence
or work on it
at another time
during the day.

it is not advisable
to do these practices
late at night
unless you want to
stay awake.

it is desirable
that you familiarize
yourself with these
exercises before you
actually do them
so that you can
perform them
in a relaxed state
with your eyes closed.

symbolic chakra exercise
BASE CENTER

sit comfortably
with your back
and neck straight,
eyes closed.

visualize at the level
of your forehead
a 2-inch by 4-inch box
full of red-orange energy.

as you inhale
through your mouth
to an 8 count,
draw the red-orange energy
down the vertebral column
to the base center.
hold it there
for a count of 16.
then exhale it
through your mouth
to an 8 count
blowing the energy
back up the vertebral column
and into the box.
observe the color
of the energy
in the box.

inhale that color
through your mouth
to an 8 count
down to the base center.
hold it there for 16.
then exhale
through your mouth
to an 8 count
blowing the energy
back into the box.
observe the color.

on the third inhalation,
draw whatever color
you found in the box
down to the base center
to an 8 count.
hold it there for 16.

then blow it out
through your mouth
to a count of 8
all around
the outside of the box
in a clockwise direction.
observe the color
around and in the box.
experience how you feel.

if the center is not clear,
repeat the sequence 3 times
and move on to
the spleen center.

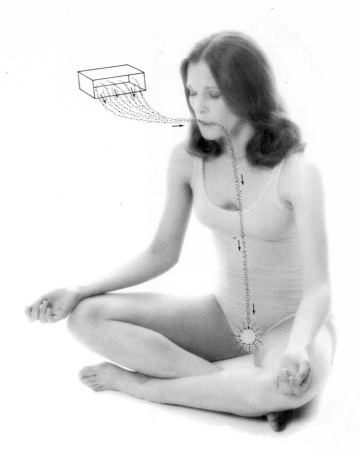

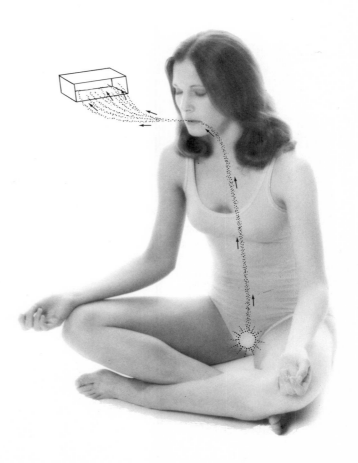

symbolic chakra exercise
SPLEEN CENTER

sit comfortably
with your back
and neck straight,
eyes closed.

visualize a glass pyramid
at the level
of your chest.
the capstone
of the pyramid
has been removed
and you can see
the four corners
that comprise the base
of the structure.
the pyramid is full
of pink energy.

draw that pink energy
through your mouth
to an 8 count
raising it up
from the four corners
and walls of the pyramid
and down
the vertebral column
to the base center.
raise this energy
to the level
of the spleen
and hold it there
for 16.
then exhale it
through your mouth
to an 8 count
blowing it up
the vertebral column,
out your mouth
and into the pyramid,
down the walls
of the pyramid
to the four corners
of the foundation.
observe the color.

inhale that color
through your mouth
to an 8 count
down to the base center.
raise it to the
level of the spleen
and hold for 16.
then, blow that energy
through your mouth
into the pyramid
to a count of 8.
observe the color

again draw that color
through your mouth
to an 8 count
down to the base center.
raise it to the level
of the spleen
and hold for 16.
then blow that energy
through your mouth
with force
to a count of 8
back into the pyramid.
as the energy comes down
into the pyramid,
the walls collapse.
observe the color, and
experience how you feel.

if the center is not clear,
repeat the sequence 3 times
and move on to the
solar plexus center.

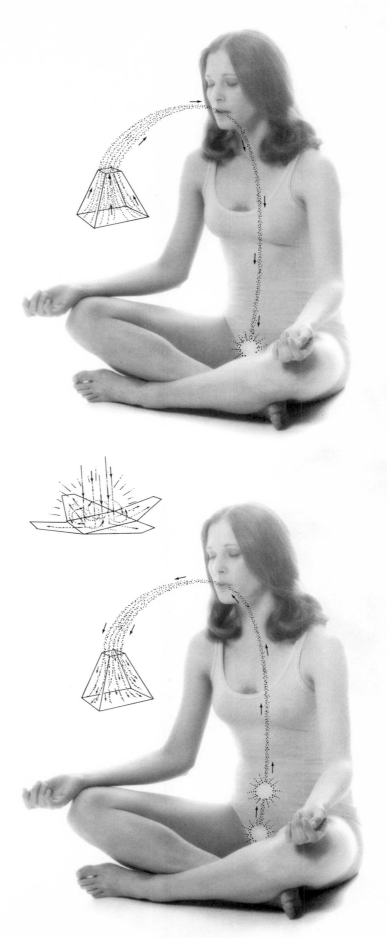

symbolic chakra exercise
SOLAR PLEXUS CENTER

sit comfortably
with your back
and neck straight,
eyes closed.

visualize an image of yourself
standing in a kelly green
disc/pool of energy.
see yourself
bend your knees
and as you start
to inhale through your mouth
to a count of 4
imagine yourself raising
this green pool
up over your head.
from this position
to a 4 count
let it turn inward
coming down the body
to the base center.
from the base center
raise this pool
to the level
of the solar plexus
and hold for 16.
then, exhale
through your mouth
to a count of 8
blowing the energy
back over your head
and down to your feet.
observe the color.

inhale that color
through your mouth
to a count of 4
bringing the pool up
over your head
and inward again
to a count of 4
down to the base center.
raise it
to the solar plexus
and hold for 16.

inhale through your mouth
to an 8 count
blowing the pool
up over your head
and back down
to your feet.
observe the color.

again, see yourself
bend down
and pick up
the color pool
as you inhale
through your mouth
raising it up
over your head
to a 4 count,
and down to
the base center
to a 4 count.
raise it to
the solar plexus
and hold for 16.
exhale
through your mouth
to an 8 count
and blow the pool
with force
straight up
over your head
into the sky.
observe the color.
experience how you feel.

if the center is not clear,
repeat the sequence 3 times,
and move on
to the heart center.

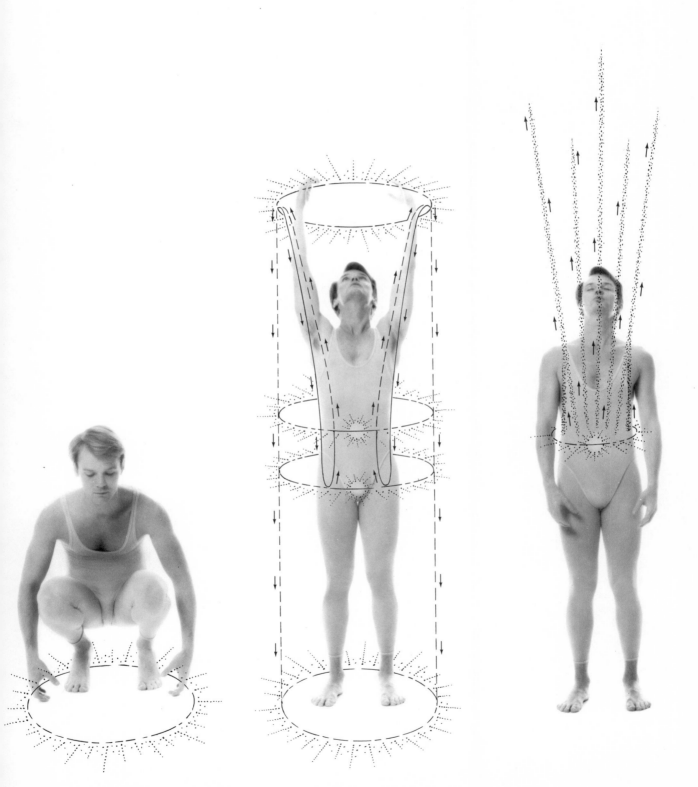

symbolic chakra exercise
HEART CENTER
———————————————

sit comfortably
with your back
and neck straight,
eyes closed.

visualize in front of you
an equilateral cross
full of yellow-golden energy.
the cross is
about the size
of your seated body.

a straw comes out
of the cross
and into your mouth.
as you inhale
through your mouth
to an 8 count,
draw all the golden energy
out of the cross
down all the vertebral column
to the base center.
raise it to the level
of the heart center.
hold it there
for a count of 16,
then blow it
through your mouth
to a count of 7
out the straw
and back into the cross.
observe the color.

again, draw that color
down to the base center
through the straw
while inhaling
through your mouth
to an 8 count.
raise it to the level
of the heart
and hold for 16.
now, with force
blow it through your mouth
to an 8 count
through the straw
back into the cross

as the energy
goes into the cross,
it hits the bottom
and that pressure
forces it up
out the two
horizontal sides
and the top
like a gushing fountain.
observe the color.
experience how you feel.

if the center is not clear,
repeat the sequence 3 times
and move on
to the throat center.

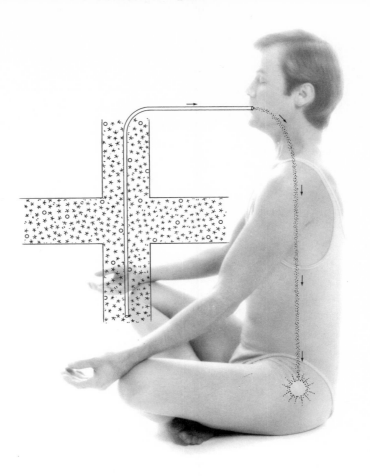

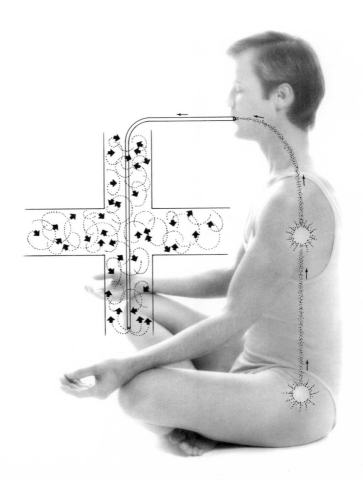

symbolic chakra exercise
THROAT CENTER

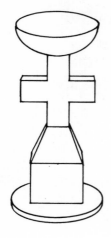

sit comfortably
with your back
and neck straight,
eyes closed.

visualize a golden chalice
composed of a circle,
a square,
a triangle,
an equilateral cross
and a crescent moon.
it is filled with
sky blue liquid light.

take hold of the chalice
above the horizontal bars
of the cross
and gently drink
the sky blue liquid,
inhaling through your mouth
to a count of 8.
gently suck it down
the vertebral column
to the base center.
raise it to the level
of the throat center
and hold it there
for a count of 16.
then regurgitate
the substance back
into the cup
while exhaling
through your mouth
to an 8 count.
observe the color.

again, gently drink
that color in and down
to the base center
while inhaling
to an 8 count.
raise it to the level
of the throat
and hold for 16
while gagging slightly.
then, regurgitate it
back into the cup
while exhaling.
observe the color.

this time, inhale
and draw that color
through your mouth
to a count of 8.
drink in the liquid energy
with gusto
and suck it down
to the base center.
raise it to the level
of the throat
where you gently
but intensely
gag on it
for a count of 16.
then regurgitate
it back into the cup
while exhaling
through your mouth
to a count of 8.
observe its color.
experience how you feel.

if the center is not clear,
repeat the sequence 3 times
and move on
to the brow center.

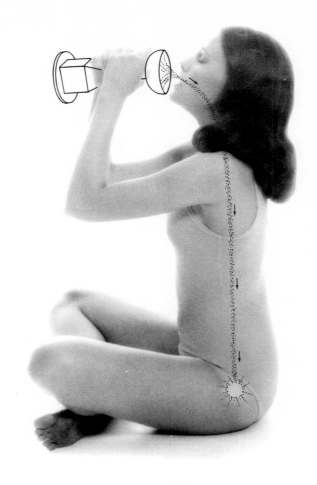

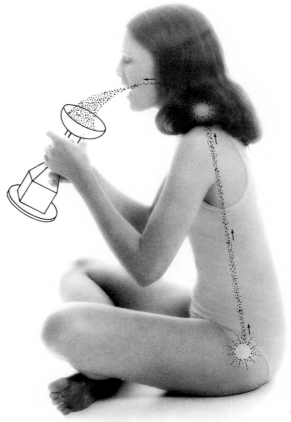

symbolic chakra exercise
BROW CENTER

———————————————

sit comfortably
with your back
and neck straight,
eyes closed.

in front of your forehead
at the level of a brow
visualize a 6-pointed star
lying on its side.
it is filled with
an indigo energy.

as you inhale
through your mouth
to an 8 count,
draw this indigo energy
counterclockwise
from the 6 points
of the star
down the vertebral column
to the base center.
raise it to the level
of the brow
and hold
for a count of 16.
then, exhale
through your mouth
to an 8 count
blowing the energy clockwise
back into the 6 points
of the star.
observe the color.

again, inhale this energy
through your mouth
to an 8 count
from the 6 points
of the star
counterclockwise.
bring it down
to the base center.
raise it to the brow
and hold for 16.
blow it through your mouth
to a count of 8

back into the
6 points of the star.
observe the color.

inhale that color
through your mouth
to a count of 8
counterclockwise
from the 6 points
of the star
and draw it down
to the base center.
raise it to the brow
and hold
for a count of 16.
then, blow it
with force
clockwise
to an 8 count
into the 6 points
of the star.
as the energy is blown
into these points
and they fill,
the energy leaps
into the air
observe the color.
experience how you feel.

if the center is not clear,
repeat the sequence 3 times
and move on
to the crown center.

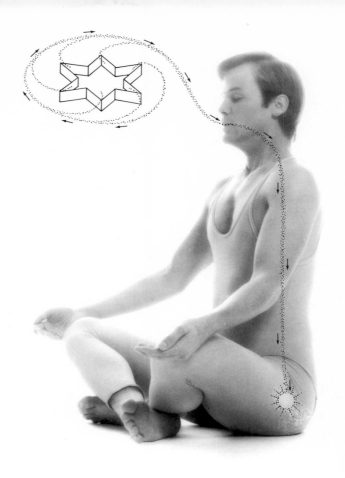

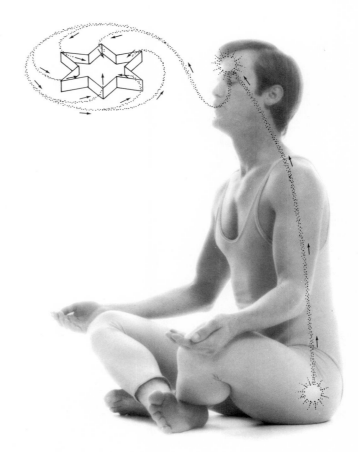

symbolic chakra exercise
CROWN CENTER

---

sit comfortably
with your back and neck
straight, eyes closed.

visualize
at the top
of your head
a closed lotus flower
filled with purple energy.

as you inhale
through your mouth
to an 8 count,
draw the purple energy
from the lotus
down through your body
and into your feet.
as the energy
is drained from it
the lotus opens completely
and remains open
until the energy returns.

now, raise the energy
from your feet
in a clockwise spiral
up your body
to the crown
and hold it there
for a count of 16.
then blow the energy
through your mouth
back into the lotus
to an 8 count
and close the lotus.
observe the color.

inhale the energy
from the lotus
through your mouth
to an 8 count
and draw it
down to your feet.
as the color is drained
the lotus opens fully.
now raise the energy
from your feet
in a clockwise spiral
up your body

to the crown
and hold it there
for a count of 16.

then close
the center of the lotus
and blow the energy
through your mouth
back into it
at a count of 8.
observe the color.

again, inhale
through your mouth
to a count of 8
drawing that color
down to your feet
as the center
of the lotus opens.
spiral the energy
clockwise up your body
to the crown.
hold it there
for a count of 16.
then, leaving the center
of the lotus open,
blow the energy
with force to an 8 count
through the open center
of the lotus
straight up
into the sky.
observe the color
and then take plenty
of time
to digest the entire
experience.

if the center
is not clear,
repeat the sequence
3 times.

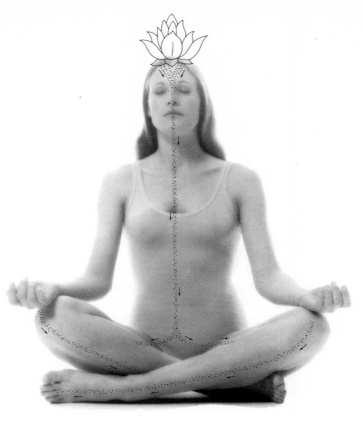

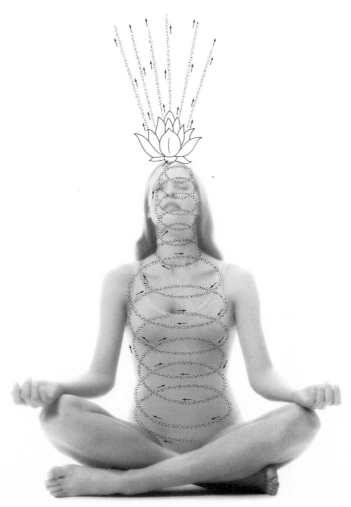

heart meditation

sitting in
meditation position
imagine a closed
golden-petaled lotus flower
at the level
of the heart.

this flower is composed
of 12 petals which
very gradually
begin to separate.
as this opening
slowly occurs,
a blue light emerges
radiating out
from the center of the flower.
as the lotus
continues to open,
the blue light expands.
take 1 to 5 minutes
for the flower
to open completely.

experience the center
totally open
emanating electric blue light.

now see a beam of white light
coming from the sky
pouring directly into
the center of the
open heart flower.

after 30 seconds
let the image go,
experience how you feel
and open your eyes.

it is important
to fuse the love energy
of the heart
with the spiritual
wisdom light.

awaken
your
sleeping
beauty

the vital root
red orange center
of procreative energy
dense latent
potent serpent power
ready to shoot
grow love
create
transmute

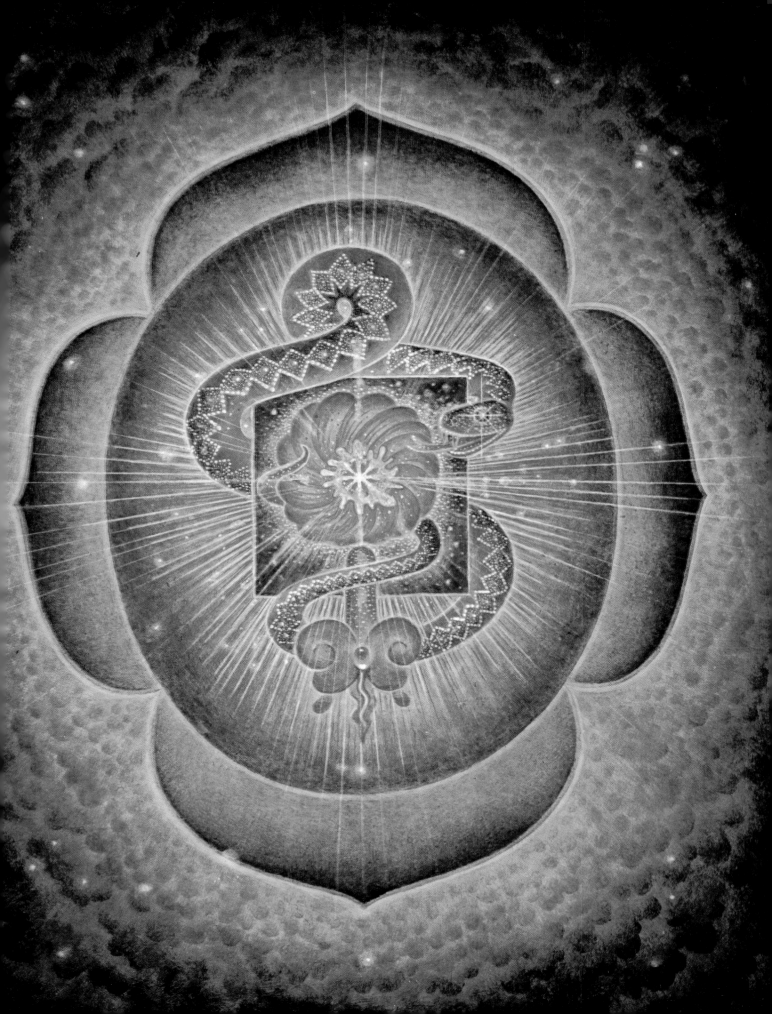

in the pink
spleen center
for purification
and health
the deep sea serpent's
rejection or protection
from anxiety
toxicity and infection

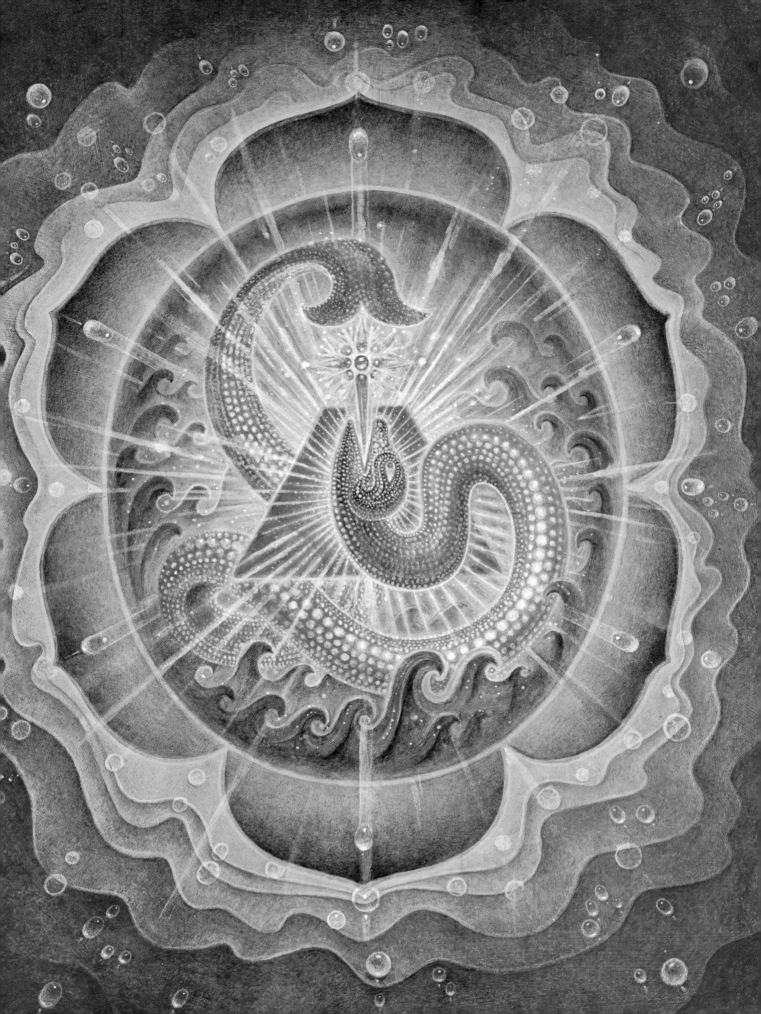

the solar plexus
fire center
for emotion and power
the green dragon
of ambition inhibition
ready to devour
or focus
open
flower

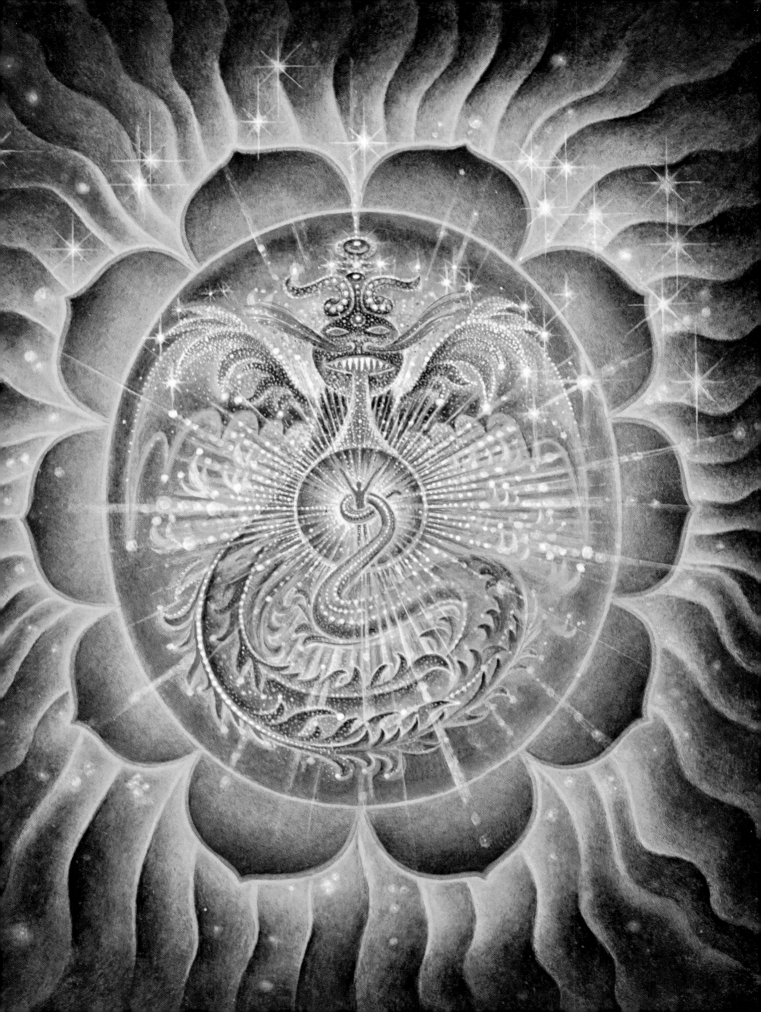

the heart
air center
for giving compassion
the snake serpent dragon
transforms
satin soft
light warms
into one
love connecting
golden sun

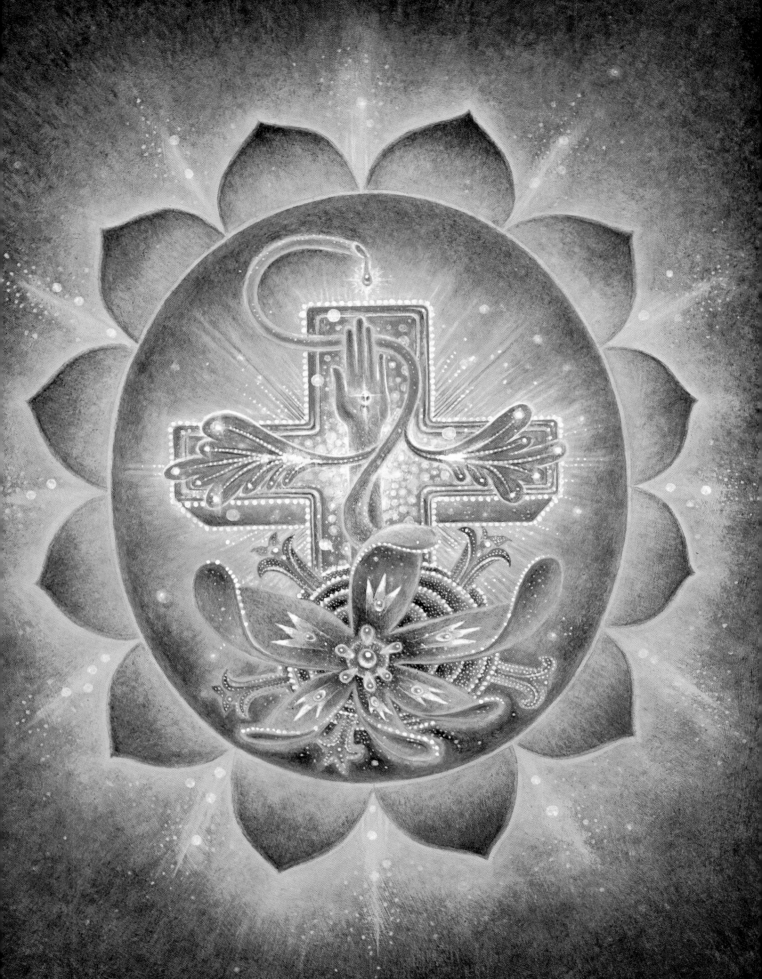

the sky blue
throat center for
creativity and
self expression
the unified
balanced
gossamer body
of elation
becomes the overflowing
cup of divine communication

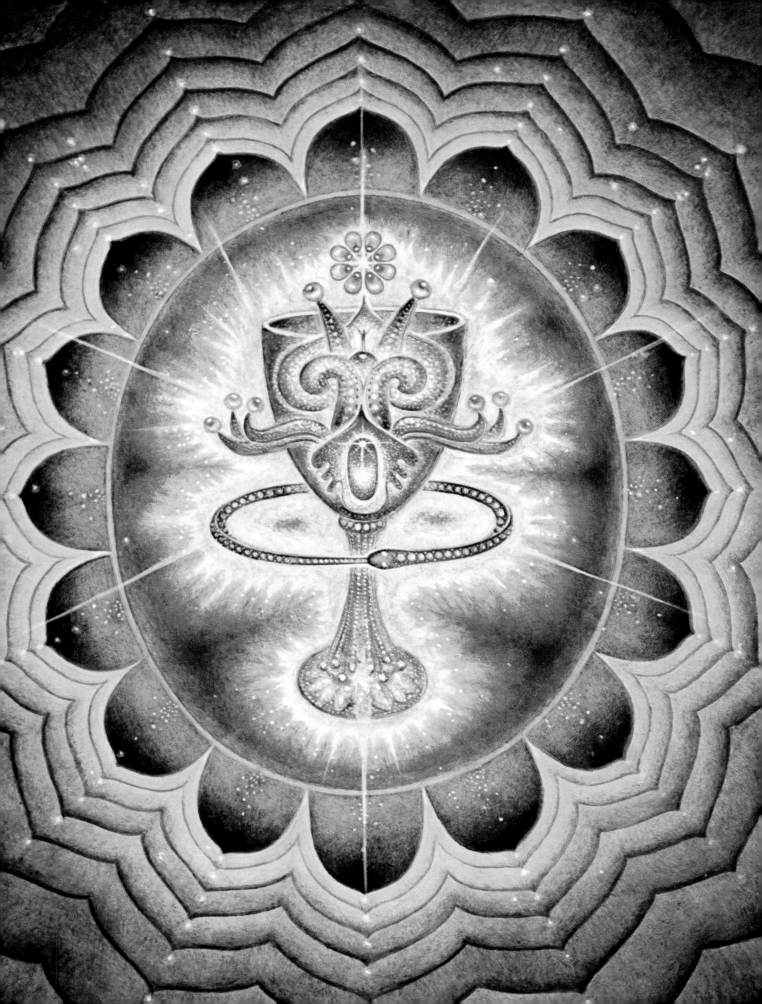

the indigo
brow center
of extrasensory
perception and
intuition
the third eye opens
in integration
ecstatic vision
and soul realization

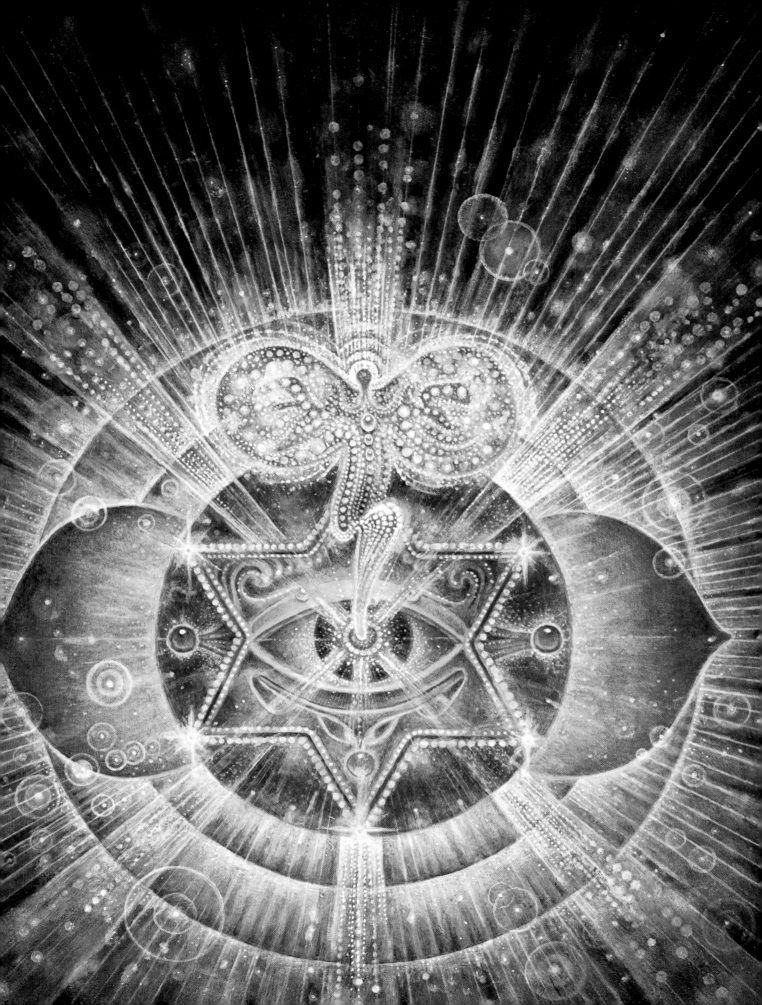

the purple
crown center
of absolute unity
silence and bliss
reality beyond duality
space
eternal

knowoneness

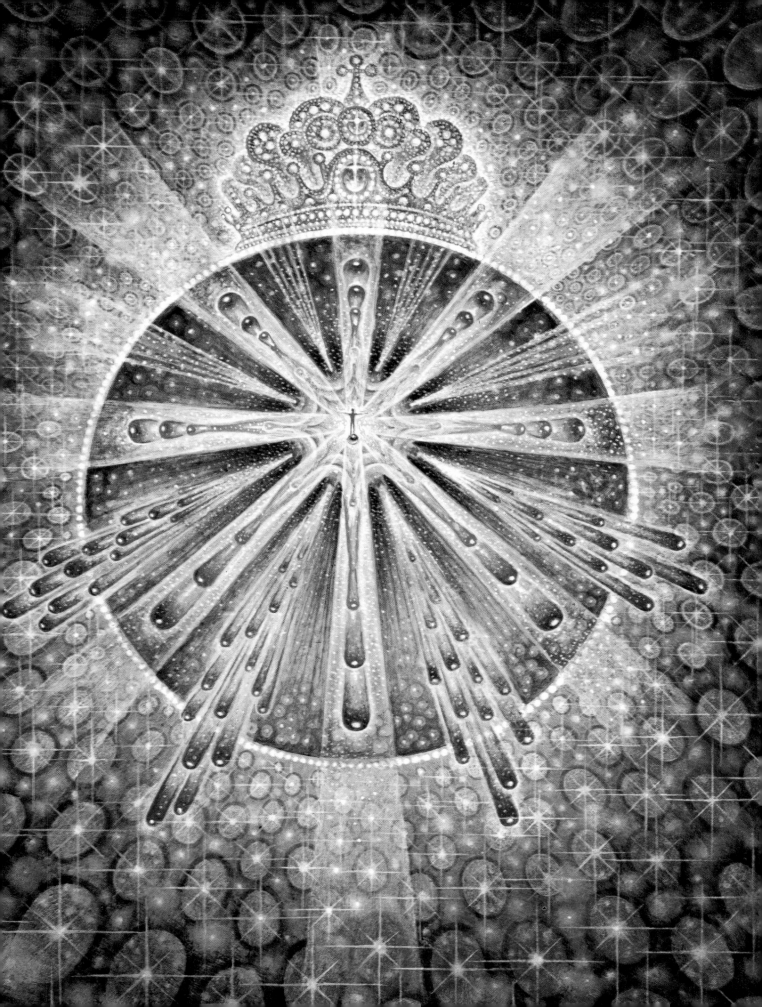

CHART OF THE SEVEN CHAKRAS

name	base center	spleen center	solar plexus	heart center	throat center	brow center	crown center
location	base of the spine	half way between pubis & navel	just above navel	center of the chest	middle of the throat	middle of the forehead	top of the head
function	sex	health	power	com-passion	creativity & self-expression	para-normal powers	libera-tion
endrocine influence	ovaries gonads	liver pancreas spleen	adrenal gland	thymus gland	thyroid gland	pitui-tary gland	pineal gland
color	red-orange	pink	kelly green	yellow gold	sky blue	indigo	purple
symbol	square	pyramid with cap-stone off	circle	cross	chalice	6-pointed star	lotus
sound	LA	BA	RA	YM	HA	AH	OM
element	earth	water	fire	air	ether		
dominant sense	smell	taste	sight	touch	hearing		
planetary influence	saturn	jupiter	mars	venus	mercury	sun & moon	
emotion	frustra-tion rage passion	anxiety well be-ing	power desire fear guilt doubt	joy grief	inspira-tion repres-sion	obses-sion ecstasy	bliss
related illness	hemorrhoids sciatica prostate ovarian uterine	diabetes cancer	ulcers gall-stones	stroke angina arthritis	thyroid flu	schizo-phrenia kidneys	psychosis

chapter 3
BREATH

breath is life
and change.

a basic connection
between the
inner/outer,
conscious/unconscious
ego and perfection.

a flowing bridge
between life
and death,
every breath
is rebirth,
inspiration,
for integration,
growth,
and re-creation.

a non-with-hold,
a letting go
of the old.
breathing is
a constant source
of energy prana
(the life force),
spirit's regeneration,
a continuous affirmation
of process,
flowing through,
weightless,
it can
in-lighten-you.

change your breathing
and you will
think/feel differently.

and this change
can be created by choice,
because breathing
is one of the few
bodily functions
that can be
voluntary
or automatic.

depression
is a deep pressing
against breathing.

it is almost impossible
to be depressed
when you are breathing
naturally.

the problem is
that most people
don't breathe normally,
that they
only half breathe,
and therefore
allow themselves
to be only half alive.

this is especially true
in a culture
which suppresses excitement
during sex and anger,
minimizing pleasure,
and maximizing anxiety.

    play it cool
    is the rule,
    and so like a fool
    we misrule.

        know
        your
        inner
        kingdom

        rather
        than
        acting
        like a
        dumb king

for breathing is power,
full/love/health,
and well being,
freeing
vitality,
giving the ability
to use your
every facility.

reverse abdominal breathing

in the reverse procedure,
the opposite
of yoga breathing.
you bring your
diaphragm in
on the inhalation,
and let the diaphragm out
on the exhalation.
it may take
a short while
to coordinate this movement,
but the results
are worth it.

temporarily
breathing through the mouth
creates more energy,
while breathing
through the nose
brings tranquility.

slow, rhythmic breathing,
facilitates
quiet and calm,
stilling the mind,
soothing the nerves,
balancing the energy
so that
in this very moment,
the inner/outer
can be experienced
as one.

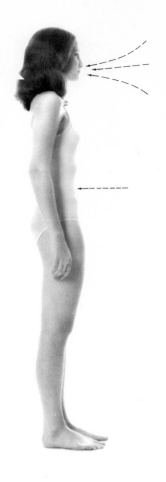

counting the breath

inhale
through your nose
to a slow
count of 8
(diaphragm comes in
on the inhalation).
hold the breath
for 4 counts.
then exhale
through your nose
to a count of 8
(diaphragm comes out
on the exhalation).
repeat this process
6 to 10 times.

regeneration breath

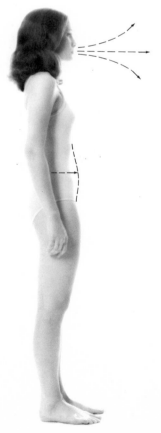

above your head see
a cloud of blue energy.
as you inhale
through your nose
(your diaphragm goes in),
fill your lungs
with this blue energy.
then, as you exhale
through your nose
(your diaphragm comes out),
see a gray substance
coming out of you
and let it go into the
empty cloud.

experience
how you feel

turn the cloud blue
and repeat the process
6 to 10 times.

expansion breath

as you inhale
through your nose
(diaphragm comes in),
imagine every cell/pore
of your body expanding.
as you exhale
through your nose
(diaphragm comes out),
imagine every cell/pore
in your body contracting.

repeat this process
6 to 10 times.

and experience
how you feel

radiating breath

fix your concentration
in the middle
of the forehead.
see a radiant jewel there.
watch and observe
what happens
as you inhale
through your nose
(diaphragm comes in),
exhale through your nose
(diaphragm comes out).
repeat this process
6 to 10 times.

raising sexual energy

sit or stand
with your back straight,
both feet
squarely on the ground.
one of your nostrils
should be closed
with your finger;
(for men,
the right nostril,
for women, the left.)

inhale through
the open nostril
and retain the air;
contract the
abdominal region
several times,
then exhale
and repeat the process
3 or 4 times.

next, inhale
through the open nostril,
and this time,
contract your anus.
while the anus is held
in a gentle,
contracted state,
imagine the energy
rising from the
base center,
and see it moving up
to the heart, throat, or
brow center.
after a
comfortable retention,
relax the anus
and exhale
through the open nostril.
repeat this part
of the process
up to 12 times.

this exercise
is a precise way
to raise and transform
emotional and
excessive reproductive
energy.

so ham
———————

inhale
as you subvocally
say SO.
exhale
as you subvocally
say HAM.

so   = that
ham = i am

repeat over and over
for an extended
period of time.

this mantra
is going on within you
all the time
as you breathe.

between breath
———————————

sit in a
comfortable position.
allow your breathng
to take over
and watch each breath.
for a while
just observe your breathing
and allow it to
regulate itself.
pay special attention
to the pauses
between the inhalation
and the exhalation,
between the exhalation
and the inhalation.
allow yourself
to deeply experience
these pauses.

these pauses
can become
experiences
of divine,
infinite space.

you are a figment
of your figment

chapter 4
CHANTING

the brain,
it appears,
has two
functionally distinct
hemispheres,
each with its own
kind of process.

the left is
rational, linear,
dualistic,
verbal,
analytical.

while the right
is holistic,
intuitive,
symbolic,
synthetic.

literally branching out
of the spinal cord,
the brain's hemispheres
can be conceived of
as the tree of knowledge,
the apple of separation
in the mind/garden of eden.

another way
of seeing
these two halves
is as yin and yang
or male and female,
the primal opposites
usually unwilling or
unable to listen
to one another
because they don't
speak the same language.

the individuation process
starts to occur,
mature,
when these two sections
begin to really
listen
to one another.
start to become sensitive
to each other,
to appreciate
that they both are
part of the same organism,
that one doesn't have to be
either rational or intuitive,
hard or soft,
passive or aggressive,
separated or united,
but that they can exist
as a whole
mind/body/soul
at the same time.

this is the
inner mystical marriage.

but the ultimate goal
is beyond
even this harmonious duality
for it is the point
at the top
of the triangle.

the totality
above the two,
the three,
the absolute unity
symbolized by
the holy trinity,
kabalistically
the tree of life.

for within the spine
and the brain
is the subtle energy body
and at its core,
the chakra system,
with its roots
in the base center,
moving up the trunk,
middle of the spine-brain,
and blossoming fully
into the
thousand-petaled lotus.

here bliss sits
forever beyond all opposites

one
with
the source sun

in the peace
that passes all understanding

pure being

without thinking
just being
radiant light love,
without
a shadow of a doubt

left
right

now

the continuous
chanting of songs
focuses the mind,
elevates
the emotions,
opens the heart,
creating,
cultivating,
the relaxed delight
of well-being.

in india
it is recognized
that the supreme
manifests
in all forms,
so songs are sung
to different manifestations
as a way
of re-identifying oneself
with the divine
within,

to be

in chanting.

shri ram
jay ram
jay jay
ram om
shari ram
jay ram
jay jay
ram ommm

sing in a
joyous tempo
repeat over and over,
eventually lower
and lower
until it disappears.

sri — great master
ram — the divine inner
aspect which pervades
all beings
jay — hail
om — essence of all

i am the peace within
i am the peace within
i am i am
i am i am
i am the peace within

this song
is a way
to reinforce
your desirable
attributes
which always exist
along with their
opposites.
it's a matter of which
you choose
to continue to
cultivate
in thought, action
and deed.

i am the _____ within
i am the _____ within
i am i am
i am i am
i am the _____ within

in each verse
put in the attitude
you wish to develop
(joy-love-bliss-
courage-harmony-strength-
humanness)
each time you sing it
you may come up
with new aspects
you wish to add/encourage.

rama rama rama
rama rama rama
rama rama rama
rama rama
ram

rama rama rama
rama rama rama
rama rama rama
rama rama
ram

repeat slowly over
and over again.

RAMA — the absolute
which pervades all beings
within and without.

thou art that
thou art that
thou art
thou art
thou art that

i am that
i am that
i am
i am
i am that

repeat over and over
at your own rhythm
and tempo.

(tat tuam asi)
that thou art
is the basic
concept/realization
behind all
yogic practices.

govinda jaya jaya
gopalala jaya jaya
govinda jaya jaya
gopalala jaya jaya
radharamana hari
govinda jaya jaya
radharamana hari
govinda jaya jaya

repeat going progressively
faster and faster.
in the end slow down
and repeat it
very slowly.

govinda — that divine aspect
which is the observer.

jaya — hail.

gopalala — another name
for krishna the joyous
irresistible aspect
of the divine within.

rada — krishna lady love
his shakti (divine energy).

radharamana — one who loves
rada and delights in
his own pure energy.

hari — one who takes
away sorrow.

listen listen listen
to my heart song
listen listen listen
to my heart song
i will never forget you
i will never forsake you
i will never forget you
i will never forsake you

repeat over and over,
fast or slow,
loud or soft.

may the long-time sun
shine upon you,
all love
surround you
and the clear light
within you
guide your way home.

remember
you are
singing
these songs
to yourself,
your own inner being.

slow down

let up
and realize

your deeper self
is there
already

chapter 5
ENERGY SOUNDS

the universe,
your mind,
is an energy generator
or degenerator.

thoughts are energy,
sounds are energy,
images are energy,
energy follows thought.

words,
sounds, and pictures
hypnotically
create your world.

how you think
affects your body,
feelings, health,
creativity,
relationships,
conflicts,
harmony, wealth.

thinking
you are a separate i,
forms your i/dentity.
believing
you are your body,
your feelings,
thoughts, possessions,
desires,
creates a restricting
i/dentification.

you are
the master
of your mind,
but you have
let the mind
master you.

you are dominated
by all of the mind clouds
with which you identify

you are free
as the sky
when you dis/identify

for example,
the idea that you
are a certain way,
that you have
all kinds of habits,
patterns and limitations,
creates
and perpetuates
this behavior.

understand that
under hypnosis,
if someone tells you
that your finger
is badly burned,
a blister will appear.

realize
in the beginning
was the word.
words are sounds,
sound is
a condensed form
of energy.
the whole world show
is a matter of energy,
every thought
an atom
constructing
your universe.

it is as if
you are not only
the actor,
but the writer,
director,
producer,
the creator
of your drama,
creating harmonious verse
or adverse reactions
to what you experience.

it's not
what happens

but what
you tell yourself

that makes it

awful

good

or bad

but ultimately,
to use another analogy,
you are
not the screen,
the motion picture projector,
or the film,
but the light, energy,
consciousness, electricity
that has a mind
and that can
watch/run the show.

you can
keep from getting lost
by constantly
remembering
who you are,
and reminding yourself
and others
that words and ideas
are models,
relative,
relatively
incomplete concepts
rather than absolute
levels of reality.

thoughts are ultimately
just noises
in your head,
a convenient, partial map,
a finger
pointing at the moon,
but not the moon.

so watch your mind;
realize that it
is the source
of all problems,
suffering, and separation,
duality, and frustration.

observe what it tells you,
what you tell yourself,
how you react,
how these thoughts move,
creating sunny spaces
or clouds
and emotional storms.

study your mind
for a brief period
and you will realize
that if anyone else
talked to you
the way your mind does,
you probably would
break the relationship
and never speak
to him again.

so then
when you get stuck
in an inner verbal pattern,
"nobody loves me,"
"i'm no good,"
"nothing ever works out,"
"god damn me,"
objectively
hear these
negative mantras,
these destructive commercials,
without reacting
to them.

in a nonattached manner,
understand
when/where
you first heard
these thoughts,
who said them,
how limited,
distorted, momentary,
and one-sided they are.

observe how
these old tapes
affect you,
and then,
if you're willing
from a
disidentified place
acknowledge their existence,
accept them,
but refuse to
go along
or be ruled by them.

then,
if you choose,
use
one of the mantras,
affirmations, or chants
in this book
to transform
the direction
of your
thought/
feelings.

for mantras are
affirmations and chants,
words, phrases,
or sometimes
sacred sounds
that evoke
a deep reaction
in, through, out
the organism.

since sound is
a highly laser-like
form of energy,
the repetition of
these vibratory patterns
can and will affect
your inner programming.

choose/use
any or all
of the following
mantras and affirmations,
repeat them out loud
or subvocally
over and over again
as you go about
your daily activity.

be sensitive as to how
each affects you.
some will be
more rewarding
than others.
use those you find
most meaningful,
and remember
in the last analysis,
you are the
final authority.

try writing them
numerous times
on a piece of paper
or in your mind's eye,
and if you
feel like it,
make up your own mantra.

so you can,
when you wish,
learn to
leave your mind
and move
into process/
experience:

a vast open space,
and ever new place
where your total being
can be.

love wisdom power
_____

i invoke the love
wisdom and power
of my higher
consciousness
to guide me
to the right activity
in the plan

to illuminate inspire
and clarify my mind
to transform transmute
and stabilize my feelings
and emotions
to energize vitalize
and heal
my physical
and vital body
so there is a normal
flow of energy
through my being
today and everyday

to attract to me
all those i can truly help
and to attract to me
all those
who can help me
in any way

this affirmation
is best used
in the morning
or before
retiring at night.

GURU OM

gu–darkness and impermanence
ru–light and permanence
om–totality

this mantra moves you
through darkness
into the light
of all totality.

repeat aloud 6 times
then subvocally
12 times
or for
as long as you like.

OM NAMAH SIVAYA

om–all
namah–i bow
sivaya–that aspect
of the divine
who promotes
the well being
of all creatures

to be sung
or spoken aloud
slowly
and then
repeated subvocally
for an extended
period of time.

cleansing affirmation

father mother consciousness
i ask
that i be cleared and cleansed
within the pure white light
the green healing light
and the purple transmuting flame

within your will
and for my highest good
i ask
that any and all disharmony
be totally removed from me
and be encapsulated
within the ultraviolet
(black) light
and cut off
and removed from me

impersonally
with neither love nor hate
i return all disharmony
to its source of emanation
decreeing that it never again
be allowed to reestablish
within me
or anyone else
in any form

now i ask
that i be placed
within a capsule of
the pure white light
and protection
and for this gift
i give thanks

use in the morning,
before retiring
or any time
during the day
when you are feeling low
or in need of
cleansing or protection.

OM MANI PUDME HUM

om—the all
mani—jeweled essence
pudme—center of the lotus
hum—everyday level of reality

this mantra
is to bring
the supreme
into this everyday level
of fully functioning
consciousness.

repeat this chant
aloud or subvocally
for an extended
period of time.

PEACE JOY PLENTY
PEACE JOY PLENTY
THE BEING WITHIN ME
IS PEACE JOY PLENTY

repeat this chant
aloud or subvocally
for as long
as you like.

unification blessing

the sons of men are one
and i am one with them
i seek to love not hate
i seek to serve
and not exact due service
i seek to heal not hurt
let pain bring due reward
of light and love
let the soul control
the outer form
and life and all events
and bring to light the love
which underlies
the happenings of the time
let vision come and insight
let the future stand revealed
let inner union demonstrate
the outer cleavages be gone
let love prevail
let all beings love

can be used
during meditation,
as an invocation,
or validation
of your relationship
to the whole.

use the name
of divine beings

SHIVA
RAM
JESUS
BUDDHA

or attributes like

LOVE
COURAGE
BLISS

and repeat
these or any sounds
you wish
over and over
for from 5
to 20 minutes.

BE STILL

AND KNOW

I AM

repeat aloud
or subvocally
as long as you wish
with an emphasis on
still, know
and I AM.

then sit in silence
and experience
your I AM.

everything's
all
light

chapter 6
ENERGY CONTACTING OTHERS

energy is continually
created and exchanged
through contact.

beings who are open,
interact, intersect,
interfuse, interlace,
interchange, interest
more than people
are who closed/
tight/isolated.

for healthy relationship
is an inter/relationship,
verbal or nonverbal
commun/i/cation.

vitality in a flow,
to and fro,
an invisible, feelable,
connecting intercourse
between energy beings,
in various ways,
on a multitude of levels.

or for that matter,
openness can become
direct contact
with any
external/internal source,
thoughts,
feelings,
food,
flowers,
work, play.
any way,
it all depends
on the degree
of separation and unity.

at the opposite extreme,
contracted,
subject/object relationships
are unconscious,
automatic, and defensive,

closed off.

not really alive
or real
because the current,
the ongoing,
ingoing, outgoing
experience/energy/feeling
is blocked off.

the excessively
defensive individual
is buying
safety and security
at the expense
of minimizing vitality
and life.

only letting
experience be
partially
or hardly at all,
continuous contraction,
suppression, and inhibition,
a trickling expenditure
of energy
with little or no return.

contact on the other hand,
for example,
between two or more
sensitive, aware,
interconnecting beings
is stimulating,
recharging, regenerating.

a perpetual,
perpetuating glow,
a flow that moves
back and forth,
that recycles,
that nourishes.
when this exchange
becomes more fully open,
there is
less and less
sense of separation.

in stillness, activity,
or conversation,
the other ultimately
becomes the self,
and the self
becomes the other,
and what is,
is.

extra/ordinary
and zen's
nothing special.

this is the symbolism
behind tantric yoga,
for the tantric sexual union
is symbolic
of this kind
of complete intimacy.

but meditative love
is only one
of many ways,
openings, to ultimately
join with
any/every/no/thing
to become,
to be,
unity,
consciousness, energy,
fully
with one's self.

in an i-thou
flowing union,
boundaries dissolve,
and you-it are one.
whether it is contact
with the sun,
the ground,
the sea,
breathing, touching,
people, emotions,
contemplation, or action,
it's all energy.

contact is some degree
of totality,
and ultimately
it can be
at/one/ment,
communion.

you become the flow.
this point is meditation,
the experience, essence,
is tantra,
realization
that you are
love, wisdom,
all.

the perfection
that is,
aways was
and always will be.

the following
meditations
on energy relationship
in this chapter
will assist you
to move
in this direction.

until at last
there is
no ego,
no other,
just energy,
consciousness, being,
the infinite
love play
of eternal delight.

energy handshake
_____

face your partner.
put your hands out
to each other
left palm up
right palm down
below and above
your partner's hands
without making physical contact,
your hands an inch or two apart.
close your eyes and feel
the energy between you.
move your hands
up and down,
closer and farther apart
and experience the
inner/outer limits
of your energy fields.
open your eyes and explore
all the possibilities
open to you.
after, discuss the experience.

energy embrace
_____

without touching,
physically
embrace each other
face to face
and remain silent
in this position
for a comfortable
period of time.
then separate
and share your experience.

feeling/calming
the energy body

have your partner
stand up
and close his eyes.
now with your hands
about one inch
from your partner's body,
explore the outline
of his energy field.
start at the head
and slowly move down,
up, and around
the neck, shoulders,
and arms,
then the torso and
upper back.
be sensitive to temperatures
and open spaces
or different kinds of
vibrations
in the field.
next do a thorough job
over the hips
and legs.
afterwards, go over
the entire body
from head down to toes,
back, front, and sides.
finish the process
by moving the hands
from the bottom
of the toes,
up the front of
the body,
over the head,
and down the back
of the body to the floor.
repeat this movement
fully, 3 times.

give your partner
a chance to experience
the results.
if you wish,
exchange verbally what the
two of you experienced
during this interaction.
then, if desired,
have your partner
do the same for you.

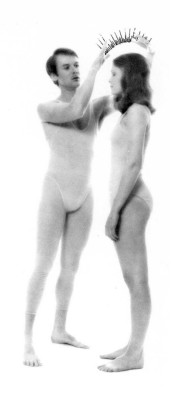

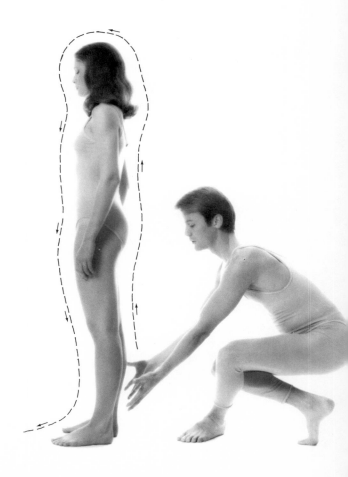

opening to gravity

stand facing your partner
and close your eyes.
allow each other
time to center
and then take your
partner's hands.

without moving
become aware of their
size, shape, and temperature.
then concentrate on the
energy flow between you.

next get in touch
with the energy pull
called gravity;
the energy that comes from
the center of the earth
which keeps you grounded,
from flying off the planet.
feel the force, its weight
and then
rather than resisting it
let it come into you.
open the bottom of your feet
and allow it to enter you.
see/feel it
as a golden energy
flowing through your feet,
melting all your
muscles, bones, nerves.
then open your ankles
and as it melts that area
let it move up
into your lower legs.
feel it flood your knees
and gently flow up
into your thighs.
let this flowing energy
wash into your hips,
through your hips
and into your lower
belly and back,
moving up into your
chest and upper back,
through your shoulders.

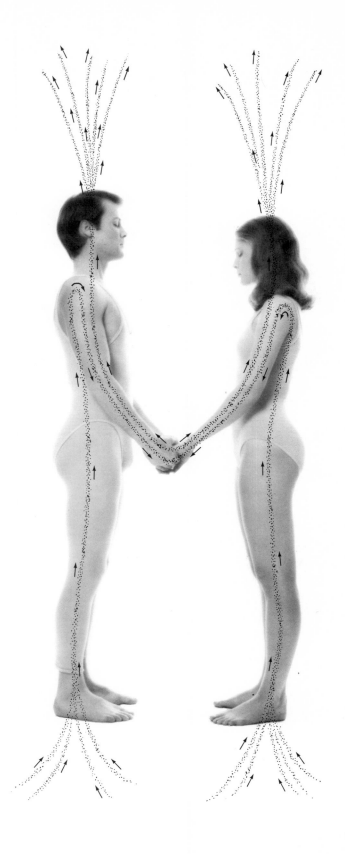

experience this energy
within you.

then let it move
down your arms,
elbows, forearms,
wrists and hands
into your partner's hands.

feel this stream
of golden energy
moving from the floor
through you,
up your body and
out your arms
into your partner's
hands, arms and body.
at the same time
experience energy
coming from your partner
into your hands and arms,
up through your shoulders
up into your neck,
jaw, cheeks, eyes, forehead,
back of the head and
out the top of your skull.
feel the energy
streaming through
and into you
from your partner
and from the ground.
hold this feeling/image
as long as you want to,
then when you feel
it's enough, let go
of your partners hands.
experience how you feel
and open your eyes.

exchange verbally
with your partner
what happened for you
during the exercise.

most of us
treat gravity
as an enemy.
in this exercise we
open to gravity
so that rather than
it being heavy,
we become light.

center touches
——————————

with eyes closed,
the person to be touched
creates a 6-inch sun
6 inches above
the top of his head.
next, he arches that sun
in front of his body
to the level of
the base of the spine.

the touching partner
visualizes a sun
6 inches above his head
and imagines that
this sun comes down
between his hands.
the person to be touched
now brings his sun
from the front of his body
into the base chakra
just in front of the spine
and sees it glow there.
the person doing the touching
brings his hands
to the level of
his partner's base center,
the right hand in front
of the body,
the left hand in back
of the base of the spine.
as the hands make contact
with the body,
the toucher's sun
fuses with the sun of
the person being touched.
both partners
see their combined suns
blazing within
the first center.

after 30 to 60 seconds,
the toucher presses his hands
gently but firmly inward
and moves his hands and sun away.
the person who has
been touched feels the
effects and then moves his
sun to the spleen center
and repeats the procedure.

continue this same
balancing, energizing contact
with your hands over
the solar plexus
and both your suns
blazing there.
repeat this process
over the heart center,
the throat center,
the brow center,
and over the crown center.
when working on the crown,
stand behind your partner
and put both hands
on the top
of his head.

when you finish,
both partners
return their suns
to the point
6 inches above
the top of the head
and allow each other time
to experience
the results.

it is desirable
to follow this procedure
with a brushdown.

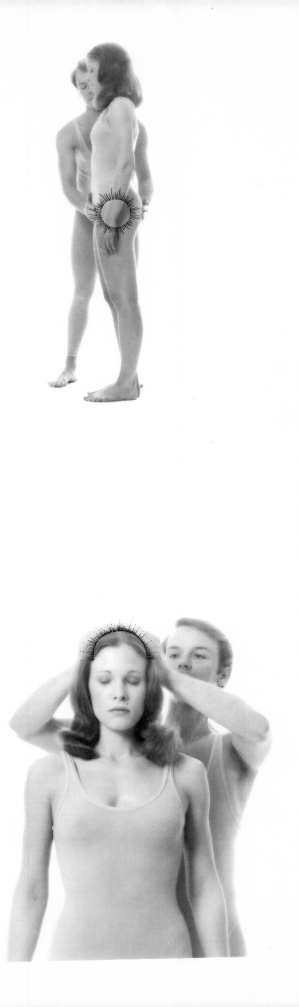

brushdown

stand behind your partner.
he closes his eyes.
put your hand on top
of his head and
stroke down the back
of his head and neck,
down the middle of the back
over the center
of the buttocks and off.

then place your hands
on top of the head again.
bring your hands
down over the outer
back of the head and neck,
down over the outer
shoulders and down the
outer back,
over the outer buttocks
and off.

place hands on the side
of the head.
gently move down over the ears
and side neck,
over the shoulders,
down the arms and hands,
over the fingers and off.

now raise your partner's arms
so they are straight out
to the side
even with his shoulders,
palms down.
place your hands underneath
his fingertips,
brush across his fingers and palms,
under his arms to the armpits
and down the side of the body
over the hips
and off.

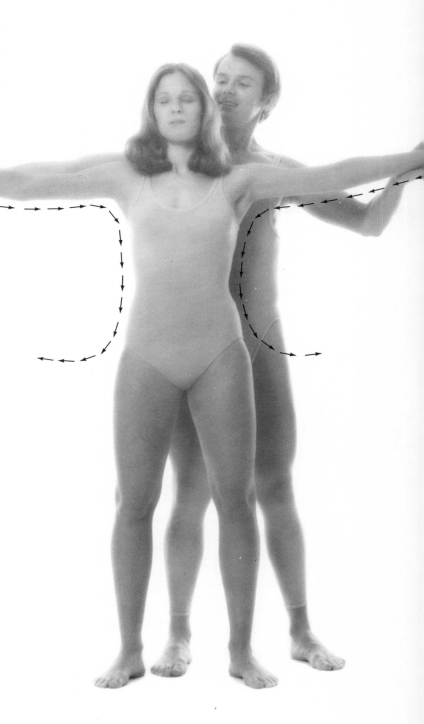

move around
to face your partner.
put your hands on top
of his head.
bring your hands
extra gently
over his face,
down over the neck,
down the center front
of the torso
to the upper pubis
and off.

place hands on top
of the outer shoulder.
bring them down
over the outer front
of the torso
to the upper pubis
and off.

raise your partner's arms
so they are straight out to the side
even with his shoulders,
palms down.
place your hands underneath
his fingertips.
brush across his fingers
and palms,
under his arms to the armpits
and down the side of the body
over the hips and off.

move to the side of your partner.
place one hand over the center
of the upper chest
and the other hand on his back
directly behind your front hand.
bring your hands over the
upper chest to the outer shoulder
down the arms, over the fingers
and off.
do this 3 times on the left
and 3 times on the right side
of your partner's body.

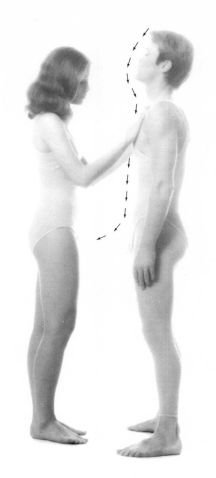

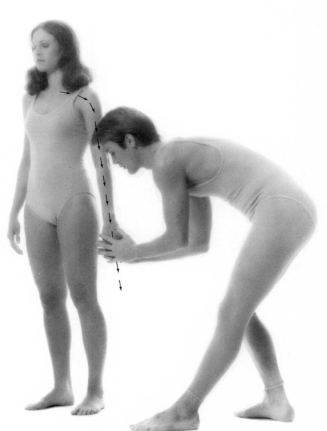

next place one hand over
your partner's front left hip,
the other hand over the buttocks
directly behind your front hand.
brush straight down
over the thigh,
the lower leg,
down over the top of the foot
and off.
after repeating this motion
3 times, do the other leg.

after, give your partner
time to experience
how he feels.

repeat each
of the strokes
3 times.
don't be heavy-handed;
use a medium gentle
wisp-like stroke
with the hand flat
over the body.
let your hand take
the shape of the place
being worked on.

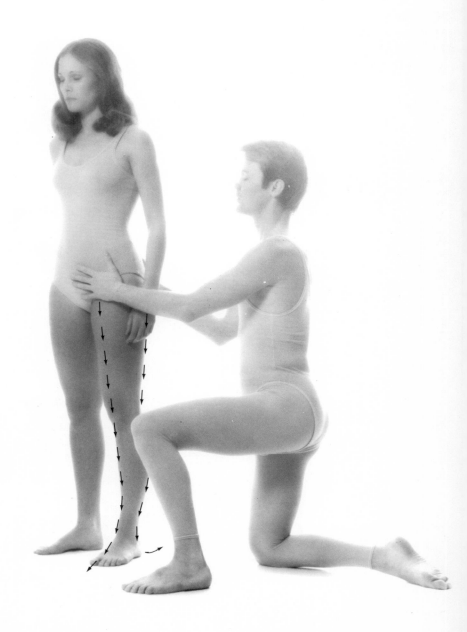

touch polarity

———————————

the person
to be worked on
lies on his/her back.
the person who
will do the touching
sits in a comfortable position
at the side of the person
lying down.

first, place your right hand
in the center of the chest
of your supine partner.
let it remain there
until you feel good contact,
the energy flowing.
next place your thumbs
on your partner's temples
at the side of the head.
the fingers of your hands
touch the ridge
on the back of the skull
where the neck joins the head.
keep a good steady pressure.
after about 30 to 60 seconds
(you can sense when it is enough)
take your hands away
and give your partner a chance
to absorb the effects
of the touch.

repeat this same time sequence
after each of the following touches.

in the next application
place your right hand
over the solar plexus
and your left hand
over the forehead,
your left thumb is on
the bridge of the nose.

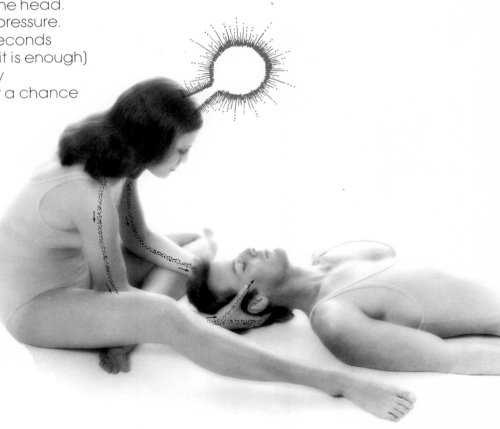

after following the time procedure,
move down to
one of your partner's legs.
let the top hand
rest on the upper middle
of the thigh.
the thumb and third finger
of the lower hand
touches the center of the ankle
just below the ankle bone.
after the allotted time,
repeat this process
over the other leg.

after an appropriate
amount of time
ask your partner to turn over.
when he/she has fully
settled on his/her belly,
make the next application
of the hands.
place your left hand
on the back top of the head
with your thumb gently pressed
into the opening
for the spine
in the skull (occiput).
the thumb and third finger
of your right hand
rest over two points
on the sacrum,
subtle indentations
to be found
approximately 4 inches
above the coccyx.

on the next touch
return the thumb and
third finger
of the right hand
to the two points
of the sacrum.
the left thumb and third finger
of the left hand
move to two points
on either side of the spine
just between the shoulder blades.

next move back to the legs.
let the upper hand
rest on the upper middle
of the thigh.
the thumb and third finger
of the lower hand
touch the center of the ankle
just below the ankle bone.
after the allotted time
repeat this process
on the other leg.

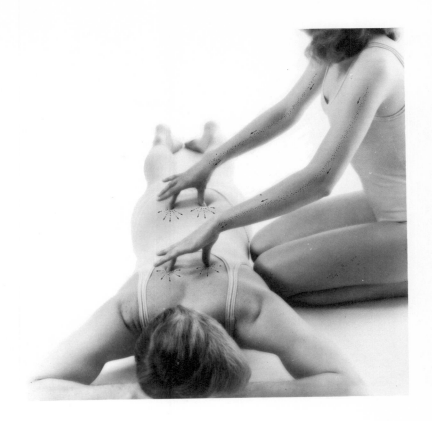

then bend the right leg
at the knee.
put the
ball of the foot
under your left armpit,
to stretch
the achilles tendon
and with your left arm,
massage the right calf.
with the right hand
gently press
all the areas of the gluteus.
repeat this process
over the opposite leg.
finally place the left hand
over the crown of the head,
the right hand
at the peritoneum
between the anus
and the genitals.

after, allow your partner
as much time as he/she needs
to digest this experience.
then if you desire,
you can discuss the experience
and/ or exchange roles

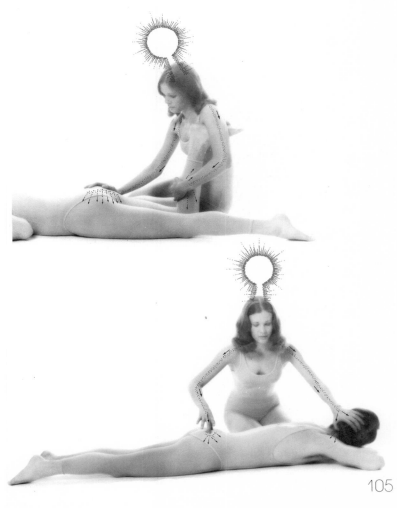

105

polarity chakras

have your partner
lie face down.

after allowing time to settle,
place your left hand
on the crown of his head.
this hand remains there
throughout the exercise.
put your right hand over
the base of his spine.
leave that hand there
for 30 to 60 seconds,
longer if necessary or desirable.

then move your right hand
over the spleen center
halfway between the pubis and navel.
after the allotted time
move sequentially to the solar plexus
just above the navel;
the heart center
in the middle of the upper back;
the throat center
at the back of the neck;
the brow center
in the middle back of the head.

now move your right hand
under the buttocks
below the base of the spine and
feel/visualize the energy
flowing freely up the spine
out all the centers
and the top of the head.

feeling/visualizing white light
on the part of the giver
and the receiver will
increase the effectiveness
of this exercise.

try combining
the exercise with
the simple polarity experience.

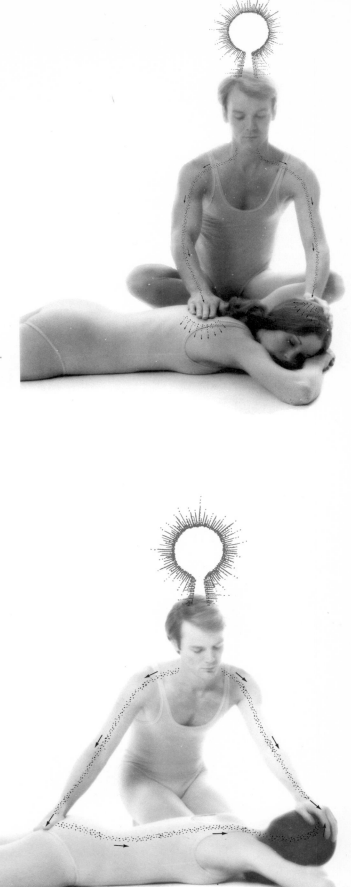

connecting chakras
_____

sit knee to knee
facing your partner.

close your eyes and
after taking time
to settle,
imagine a white light sun
in your base center,
your partner does the same.
when this sun is
shining brightly within you,
visualize it beaming out
toward your partner;
your partner does the same.
as you continue to
shine out toward your partner
imagine/feel his/her energy
emanating toward you.

after about 30 seconds,
let this energy contact
remain on its own,
and move up to and repeat
this process in the spleen chakra.
in time move up each center
one by one,
until you are connected
in all of the chakras.
see/feel this contact,
all the centers
connected and beaming,
for 30 to 60 seconds.
then let the image fade,
experience how you feel
and open your eyes.

this procedure
can be done
laying on your side
next to your partner
in bed.

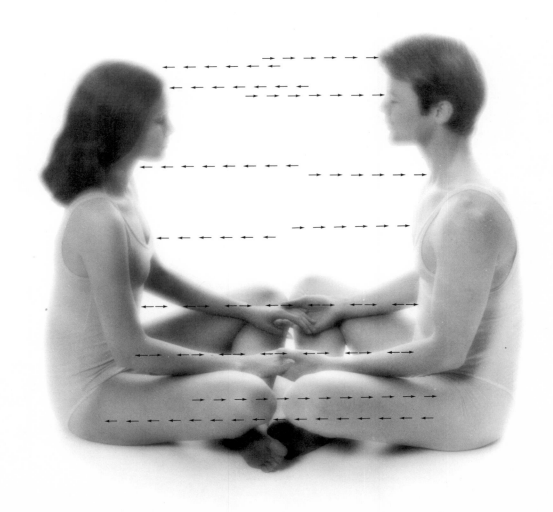

there's no
you or me
there's
just we e e e e e e e e e e e e e e e e e e e e e e e e e e e

chapter 7
ENERGY HEALING

health is bliss,
wholesomeness,
flowing energy,
in harmony
with totality.

a well
organized organism
works with
integrated integrity
as each part relates
and operates
with the whole.

a continuously
rebalancing,
connecting,
exchanging,
overlapping
interrelationship
with all/
every aspect of
environment/other/
mind/body/soul,
a complete whole.

healing
is the process
of un-dam-ing,
rebalancing,
and/or boosting
of the energy
throughout
the organism.

a transfer,
transformation,
or removal of energy
from one force field
or a series of
force fields
to another,
be it magnetic,
chemical, physical,
electrical, surgical,
emotional, or psychic.

for ultimately
most all dis/ease
is caused
by a blackage
or imbalance
in the core/energy body.

usually this is
brought about
because one part
of the system
tries to dominate
the organism
at the expense
of other parts
or the whole.

symptoms are then
usually the expression
of a subordinate part
or parts
that are in conflict—
that don't accept
the dominant direction,
the life style
that is
generally being pursued.

in gestalt therapy terms,
it is the classical
top dog/under dog conflict,
one part of you
is saying to
another part of you:
"you're holding me too tight,"
"you're putting me under
too much pressure,"
"stop trying to control me,"
"let me be."

a great deal of physical
and psychological distress
is the result
of these
seemingly weaker aspects
not being allowed
to really express themselves.

left with no outlet,
they use their power
to communicate
through discomfort.

at first they speak softly
through minor
aches and slight symptoms.
but not being heard,
they increase the volume
of their voice
through greater pain
and intermittent
malfunction.

if they continue
to be ignored,
they will cause
serious breakdown
or illness,
and eventually
if you refuse to
listen to them,
they will kill you.

once again,
balance
is a primary factor;
for if you either do
too much
or express too little,
and the body
or various parts,
nerves, glands,
muscles become
chronically tense,
frozen under overstress,
the flow of energy
is blocked,
and the result
is that some symptom
or malfunction appears
in a structurally weak
or symbolic area.

healing, then,
is a transformation,
a return to balance
and flow,
a continuing to
appropriately
open and grow,
to know,
to experience
your process/being.

ideally,
healing will be done
in a feeling, compassionate,
nonpersonal, objective way
where the healer
and the person
to be healed
move out of the way
and allow
the wisdom current
of the universe
to flow through them.

not acting
but having the
knowledge and faith
to allow the energy
to move through;
not creating limitations
but becoming receptive,
open channels
through which
infinite energy
is allowed to move,
to improve,
because ultimately
there's nothing to do
except to assist,
direct, and allow,
to lend a helping hand,
aiding your being
to heal itself.

now understand
all forms of healing
or therapy,
regardless of the system
or orientation, have
three basic ingredients:
suggestion, belief, and
energy transformation.

in every healing situation,
there is,
implicit or explicit,
the suggestion,
be it through
training, uniforms,
degrees, or ritual,
that the person
or practitioner
has the power
and the ability
to create a change.

second, there must be
a conscious
or unconscious belief
on the part
of the participants
that the patient
will get better.

finally, and most important,
there must be
a transfer or exchange
of energy.

if any of these elements
are missing
in any form of therapy,
usually there will be
little or no results.

in the following chapter,
we will be
primarily concerned
with self healing.
it is important
to realize,
as you do
these exercises,
that excessive skepticism
or expectations
will create minimal
results.

if you can be
open and receptive,
you will find
these different methods
for wholeness,
synthesis,
self regulation,
cleansing,
rebalancing,
and deconditioning
simple, effective
ways to erase old tapes,
to equalize the
energy organism,
to keep it clear,
in a constant state
of flowing,
harmonious wholeness
that is health
and holiness.

earth air fire water

with your eyes closed,
relax and visualize
an image of yourself
moving toward a
body of water.
have that image stop,
turn and face you.
take a good look at it.
now have the image turn
toward the body of water
and become identified
with the image.
as you move
toward the body of water
notice that
there is a large
pile of clay
as well as a
pile of wood nearby.
take some clay
and using the water
to soften
and smooth the clay,
build a statue of yourself.
it can be any size
and in any style you wish.
as you construct it,
it may change
or take on a shape
different than
what you intended to build.
allow this
unconscious process
to take over.

when you feel
you are finished
stop and take a look
at the work.
then with the water
smooth it out and
add any details or
final touches.
when you have finished,
again look at the whole statue.
now go to the wood
and begin to pile it
under and around
the statue.

then, light the wood
and watch the statue
burn in the flames.

out of the smoke,
or from the cracking statue
something desirable
will emerge
and circle above in the air.
if it is something
acceptable to you,
allow it to enter
and become
part of the image.
now see the image
walking toward you.
when it is a few feet away,
ask it to stop
and take a look at it.
observe how it looks.
see if it is different
than before,
then allow it to merge
with you.
take time to experience
how you feel.
open your eyes.

this visualization
may be done
every day.
it is a way
to integrate and balance
the 4 basic elements,
to purify your self,
to not get stuck
in any image,
to allow latent
constructive forces
to emerge.

after experiencing it
a few times
it can be done
very quickly,
without diminishing
the results.

tantrum meditation

for 5 or 10 minutes
breathe randomly in and out
through the nostrils
while walking around the room.

for 5 to 10 minutes
move around the room
in whatever manner
you are moved to.
allow your arms and legs
the freedom to take over.
allow the sounds within you
to do the same.
move as fast or as slow
as you need to,
make as much or as little
noise in whatever way
you need to.

for 5 or 10 minutes
with your arms raised,
elbows even with your head,
jump up and down,
landing on your heels..
each time you come down,
make the sound WOO.

after, take some time
to allow this experience
to settle within you.
it may bring out
suppressed feeling aspects
of chaos which
need to be let out
so that your energy
can flow free.

a way to release/relieve
tension/pent-up emotion
and deep chronic
nagging discord.

lost treasure
_____

find a comfortable place
to sit or lie down.
close your eyes and
allow yourself time
to deeply relax.

visualize yourself standing
at the edge of a
clear, calm lake
on a warm, sunny day.
feel the peace
of the location
and the warmth of the sun.

just in front of you
there is an open boat
in the water
full of big, soft pillows.
see yourself lying down
in the boat
as it drifts toward the
center of the lake.
like the boat floating
on the water
experience yourself floating
on the pillows,
and completely relax.
when you reach the
center of the lake
imagine yourself
sitting up in the boat
and finding
a magic diamond pendant
which you put
around your neck.
it will protect you
from any harm and
give you magical powers
like the ability to
swim easily,
breathe under water
and have great strength.

now, dive into the water
and swim down to the bottom.
(remember the diamond
if you should need it.)

after a short search
you will find
an old treasure chest
containing something valuable,
a positive attribute
that you possess
but are not in touch with.
bring the chest
to the surface.
if it is heavy
use your magic diamond.
swim to the shore and
open the treasure chest.
if it is locked,
use the diamond
to open it.
if you don't understand
what emerges
from the chest,
it will speak to you
and your diamond
can help you understand.

after you have determined
what the aspect represents,
decide if you
would like to again have
this treasure as a
conscious aspect of yourself.
if this is what you wish,
stand up and face the sun.
either embrace the aspect
or hold it up to the sun.
see the part melt into you.
after you experience this union
hold the magic diamond
up to the sun
and let it merge and
become a conscious part of you.
finally, see the sun
enter and merge with you.
after, take time to
absorb this entire experience
and then open your eyes.

this can be done
over and over again
to re/establish contact
with hidden or disowned
aspects of your self.

erasing doors

find a quiet place
to sit or lie down.
close your eyes
and allow yourself
to relax completely.

now, see an image of yourself
walking into a house
and down a long corridor.
you will pass 3 doors
on your right
and 3 doors
on your left.
notice there is a label
on each door to your left,
a word or two
that describes
what is behind it.
take note of each
as you walk by.
these labels are not
created by your conscious mind
but rather they are
meaningful areas your
unconscious wishes you
to explore.
now return to stand
in front of the door
which is most intriguing
or meaningful to you.
before opening the door
surround yourself
from head to toe in
a circle of white light
for protection and
then go into the room.
see/feel and be aware
of what you find
in the room
from a dis/identified
point of view.
you may find past feelings,
events, old relationships
or associations.

experience whatever is there,
no matter how undesirable
or painful
but from an unattached perspective.
watch as you allow
any emotional reactions
to take place.
stay with the experience
until all excessive feelings
have been discharged.
now bring in a bright light
to illuminate the room
allowing you to see
details that did not show up
under ordinary light.
observe/experience and allow
these situations to discharge.
when nothing new seems to emerge,
flood the entire area
with cleansing white light
erasing everything in the room.
come out of the room
and explore
the other 2 rooms
or walk over to the right
side of the corridor.
this time consciously
put a label on each
of the 3 doors,
subjects like sex, anger, fear,
love, work or relationships.
choose the one
you most wish to explore.
first envelop yourself
in a circle of white light
for protection,
and enter the room.
as you did on the other side,
see/experience what is there
from a dis/identified space,
then bring in more light
so that you can see
with clarity
all the details.

when you feel
nothing new is emerging,
flood the room
with white light
erasing everything that is there.
then walk out of the room.
(you can experience each
of the doors in turn
if you wish.)
when you feel finished
return down the corridor
and out of the house
through the door
by which you entered.
after, take some time
to digest your experience
and then open your eyes.

often during this exercise
you will see
pictures of the past,
remember old feelings
or associations.
by letting these situations
discharge without
being attached
you will finish them.

this process
can be used
to clear karma
at the end of each day
by taking your problems
or upsets
through the rooms
in the above way.

heal thyself

if you have an illness,
symptom or problem
you do not understand,
find a quiet place
and lie down on your back.
close your eyes.
for 5 to 10 minutes
imagine you are lying
at the edge of the seashore.
your feet are facing
the water.
as you inhale each breath
imagine the water from the ocean
washing over and through
your body
relaxing, cleansing and
re-energizing you.
as you exhale
the water washes down
and out the back
of your body
removing all toxins,
waste and fatigue.

when you are
deeply relaxed
visualize yourself
in a clearing
surrounded by a forest.
experience the color, smell,
and feeling of the area
as intensely as possible.
then, from the trees
that surround the clearing
a figure of a person,
animal or being will emerge.
it represents
the symptom or problem.
have a dialogue with this image:
ask who it is, what it wants,
and what it can tell you
about your difficulty.

it may be mad or shy at first
and refuse to speak.
it is your task
to convince it
that you are genuinely
interested in learning
its needs.
(see if you can really listen
to what this aspect of yourself
is trying to communicate.)

ask any questions you wish
and be really open
to hearing the answers.
usually this being
is talking for a part of you
that you have ignored.
often it will tell you something
you don't want to know
but need to hear.
many times it will represent
your childlike nature
wanting you to relax, play
and enjoy life more.

whatever its needs are
see if you can accept them.
if you are willing
to do what is asked,
let the being know that.
ask if it is willing
to meet you the following day
for 10 minutes
or perhaps every day for a week.
if you make any appointments
with the figure
be sure to keep them,
or you will destroy
the relationship/communication
you have established.

when you feel finished,
thank the being for coming
and watch it disappear
into the forest.
then, when you are ready,
let all the images fade
and open your eyes.

this interaction may
not only dis/solve
your symptom
but provide you
with a friend/guide
who will assist you
in various other aspects
of your existence.

healing inside/out
————————————

close your eyes
and become comfortable.

slowly scan your body
for points of pain
or excessive tension.
when you find an area
that needs some attention,
place your hand there.
experience how that
place feels.
let your hand rest there
as you begin to visualize
the color, texture,
and quality of that area.
next see an image of yourself
getting smaller and smaller
until it is the right size
to walk around inside your body.
now see that image
moving through your body
to the place
that is to be investigated.
explore that area;
find out what it needs,
what you as that image
can do to create more ease
and harmony there.
stay as long as you need to
and then open your eyes.

repeat this process
as many times as necessary,
and then if desired,
move to other areas.

visual healing

in bed at night
just before you
go to sleep
or any time
during the day,
close your eyes
and relax.

see the number 5.
let it fade
and create it
two more times.
do this same process
with the numbers
4-3-2-1 and 0.
after you have
made the 0 three times,
see yourself standing
in the center of the 0
in perfect health.
experience yourself
with as much detail as possible.
then imagine yourself
doing all of the things
you would be able to do
in perfect health.
see yourself doing
all these things as completely
as possible, see yourself
successfully and joyously
doing each task until
you go to sleep.

do not see the injury
getting better,
this gives energy
to the problem.
rather, see the healing
as already having
taken place.

you are
perfect
at this
very moment
you are perfect
and you
have always
been so
yet you go on
seeking
for perfection
because your mind
tells you that
you are incomplete.
you define yourself
as incomplete
as a seeker
and because
of this definition
you never
really experience
your real
buddha nature
buddha is
one who finds
who is enlightened
who attains
who is total
while you
live in
the constant hope
that this book
this seminar
this guru
will be the answer

there is no answer
because ultimately
there is no question
questions and answers
are the mind's game
so that you
cannot attain
it is the game
of postponement
some day
in the future
my enlightenment
will come

and so you go on
pursuing goals
desires happiness
but when
you finally get
what you think you want
that is not it
or you don't want it
anymore

here and now
in this very moment
you are one
with the sun
air ground sky sea
free
totally
completely
utterly

only you
don't believe that
you don't think
this is true
and that very you
is what keeps you
from realizing

for realization
is giving up
and down
in and out
any mental knowing
of what it's
all about

letting go
becoming the flow
becomes the glow
completely being
the son/daughter
of cosmic life
here to know
beyond knowing

it's your
forever now
perfect
self

117

perfection is
your very core

but you
seldom realize it
anymore

don't identify
with the changing
rearranging
outer duality

you are bliss

consciousness

love's
everlasting
reality

so breathe deep
and open
the rainbow door

enter the bright diamond
that is the other shore

dance to the inner lights
soar to the inner heights
bask in the inner delights
warm sun days without nights

in the peace within
the outer war

for perfection is
your very core

you

god

it

BIBLIOGRAPHY

Assagioli, Roberto, M.D., *The Act of Will,* Viking Press, 1973.

Assagioli, Roberto, M.D., *Psychosynthesis: A Manual of Principle and Techniques,* Psychosynthesis Research Foundation, 1965.

Atkinson, William W., *Thoughts Are Things,* L.A. Fowler & Co., 1912.

Bailey, Alice A., *Esoteric Psychology: A Treatise of the Seven Rays* (Vols. 1 and 2), Lucis Publishing Co., 1942.

Campbell, Joseph, *The Mythic Image,* Princeton University Press, 1974.

Garrison, Omar, *Tantra,* Academy Editions, 1972.

Harding, D.E., *A Contribution to Zen in the West,* Harper & Row, 1972.

Huxley, Aldous, *The Perennial Philosophy,* Harper & Bros., 1945.

Iohari, Harish, *Leela,* Coward, McCann & Geoghegan, Inc. 1975.

Keges, Ken, Jr., *Handbook to Higher Consciousness,* Living Love Center, 1972.

Krishnamurti, Jiddu, *Freedom From the Known,* Harper & Row, 1969.

Leadbeater, C.W., *The Chakras,* Theophysical Publishing House, 1968.

Metzner, Ralph, *Maps of Consciousness,* MacMillan Co., 1971.

Mishra, Rammurti S., *Fundamentals of Yoga,* Julian Press, Inc., 1959.

Oyle, Irving, *The Healing Mind,* Celestial Arts, 1975.

Rajneesh, Bhagwan Shree, *The Book of Secrets,* Harper & Row, 1974.

Ramacharaka, Yogi, (name assumed by William W. Atkinson), *Raja Yoga or Mental Development,* The Yogi Publication Society, 1905.

Ramacharaka, Yogi, *Science of Breath,* The Yogi Publication Society, 1905.

Rawson, Phillip S., *Tantra, The Indian Cult of Ecstasy,* Avon, 1973.

Rendel, Peter, *Introduction to the Chakras,* Samuel Weiser, 1974.

"Three Initiates," *The Kybalion,* The Yogi Publication Society, 1908.

Watts, Alan W., *The Wisdom of Insecurity,* Pantheon, 1951.

acupuncture a traditional chinese healing technique in which fine needles are placed in key points on the body to free congestion and balance energy

akido a defensive japanese martial art; its goal is neither defeat nor injury but centered-ness and learning to use the momentum of your opponent's energy

aquarian the age officially begins approximately the year 2000 to bring a period of inventions, brotherhood, enlightenment, spiritual rebirth and peace.

astral spaces the timeless, materialess space of dreams and out-of-the-body experience

aura a series of energy fields that surround the physical body

chakra a wheel or vortex acting as a sending/receiving center for cosmic energy

esoteric secret knowledge that is not for public disclosure

etheric the subtle energy vibration or field within and around the gross physical body

exoteric knowledge no longer belonging to an inner circle of disciples or initiates

holistic the whole equals more than the sum of the parts. an approach to human behavior based on the view that man is a unified organism and that every inner/outer aspect affects the whole

homeostatic a state of more or less temporary psycho/physiological equilibrium or balance

kabalistic (kabala, cabala) a pragmatic, occult philosophy based on an esoteric interpretation of the hebrew scriptures

karma the law of cause and effect; past thoughts, habits, and behavior create present circumstances. karma yoga is the path of non-attached service.

kirlian a method of photographing the aura (energy field) of organic objects (example: leaves, fingertips)

kundalini the basic earth energy which resides in the first chakra. this latent serpent power can be activated upward, unfolding towards spiritual illumination

lotus an aquatic asiatic plant that symbolizes openness, enlightenment and non-attachment, sometimes used to describe the chakras

mantra sacred words or sounds which when repeated affect a person's energy levels and state of consciousness

meditation position a seated position in which the back and neck are straight, the eyes lowered or closed and the hands placed in a comfortable position

meridians energy paths which flow through the body connecting various acupuncture points or organs

piscean an age of restriction, limitation, individualism and materialism which began approximately 2000 years ago

prana the vital essence energy within food, air plants and man

satori a state of spiritual enlightenment found through the practice of zen buddhism

t'ai chi ch'uan a holistic chinese system of health-giving balancing movement exercises rooted in the philosophy of taoism

tantra an unorthodox yogic method for experiencing total fusion with the universe. Its techniques often include the utilization and transmutation of sexual energy

zen a japanese form of buddhism which uses nature, simple everyday tasks, meditation and non-sense questions to create an atmosphere where instantaneous enlightenment can occur